Clinical Canine and Feline Respiratory Medicine

Clinical Canine and Feline Respiratory Medicine

Lynelle R. Johnson, DVM, MS, PhD, Diplomate ACVIM
(Small Animal Internal Medicine)

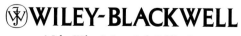

WILEY-BLACKWELL

A John Wiley & Sons, Ltd., Publication

Edition first published 2010
© 2010 Blackwell Publishing

Blackwell Publishing was acquired by John Wiley & Sons in February 2007. Blackwell's publishing program has been merged with Wiley's global Scientific, Technical, and Medical business to form Wiley-Blackwell.

Editorial Office
2121 State Avenue, Ames, Iowa 50014-8300, USA

For details of our global editorial offices, for customer services, and for information about how to apply for permission to reuse the copyright material in this book, please see our website at www.wiley.com/wiley-blackwell.

Authorization to photocopy items for internal or personal use, or the internal or personal use of specific clients, is granted by Blackwell Publishing, provided that the base fee is paid directly to the Copyright Clearance Center, 222 Rosewood Drive, Danvers, MA 01923. For those organizations that have been granted a photocopy license by CCC, a separate system of payments has been arranged. The fee codes for users of the Transactional Reporting Service are ISBN-13: 978-0-8138-1671-5/2010.

Library of Congress Cataloging-in-Publication Data

Johnson, Lynelle R.
  Clinical canine and feline respiratory medicine / Lynelle R. Johnson.
    p. ; cm.
  Includes bibliographical references and index.
  ISBN 978-0-8138-1671-5 (pbk. : alk. paper) 1. Respiratory organs–Diseases. 2. Dogs–Diseases.
3. Cats–Diseases. I. Title.
  [DNLM: 1. Dog Diseases–therapy. 2. Respiratory Tract Diseases–veterinary. 3. Cat Diseases–therapy.
4. Clinical Medicine–methods. SF 992.R47 J67c 2010]
  SF992.R47J64 2010
  636.089′62—dc22
                                                                              2009049308

A catalog record for this book is available from the U.S. Library of Congress.

Set in 10/12pt Sabon by Aptara® Inc., New Delhi, India
Printed in Singapore by Markono Print Media Pte Ltd

With special thanks to the clients and patients who have furthered my knowledge of respiratory medicine and fueled my passion for discovery. I remain indebted to my mentor Brendan McKiernan for all that he has taught me over the years.

Contents

Preface

Management of small animal patients with respiratory disease is challenging, in part because clinical signs of disease can appear similar across a large number of respiratory disorders. In addition, respiratory signs can mimic those caused by cardiac or systemic diseases, and respiratory disorders can develop secondary to these diseases. I believe that localizing disease through a comprehensive physical examination, acquiring a thorough appreciation of the most current and appropriate respiratory procedures, understanding respiratory therapeutics, and using a resource that offers descriptions of the most common respiratory syndromes are all important for making us better diagnosticians and clinicians in respiratory medicine. The goal of this textbook is simple. It is to impart that knowledge in a logically developed, easy-to-read, and well-indexed manner from the perspective of a clinician whose first love is respiratory medicine and one who is fortunate to subspecialize in this aspect of internal medicine. Throughout this book, I have organized the text for the busy practitioner wanting to practice at "the cutting-edge" of veterinary medicine and for the veterinary student looking for a thoughtful integration of clinically relevant anatomy, physiology, and disease.

I approached this task recognizing that all the comprehensive medicine textbooks contain excellent chapters on respiratory disorders. This textbook aims to provide an authoritative, cohesive, and complete discussion of all the elements needed to diagnose and treat small animal respiratory diseases specifically in a user-friendly, single-author volume. The first section deals with the common presenting signs for patients with respiratory disease: nasal discharge, loud breathing, cough, tachypnea, and exercise intolerance. This is intended as a quick reference for immediate localization of the site of disease in order to guide diagnostic investigations. The next section contains detailed how-to descriptions of all those important diagnostic methods. I then devote an extensive chapter to therapeutic options. All medical options are covered in detail with canine and feline dose rates for the drugs that I find useful in the management of simple and complex respiratory diseases. The remainder of the book has thorough explanations of individual diseases divided into chapters dealing with disorders of the nose, airways, lung parenchyma, pleura, and pulmonary vasculature. Each chapter follows the same easy-to-read order with diseases subdivided by etiology: structural, infectious, inflammatory, and neoplastic disorders.

I hope that this textbook will instill confidence in students and practitioners as they identify and manage respiratory conditions in dogs and cats.

Lynelle R. Johnson

Acknowledgments

I am indebted to my colleagues in medicine, radiology, cardiology, critical care, clinical pathology, and pathology at the University of California, Davis, who provided me with the intellectual stimulation, collegiality, and wisdom to create this book. Special thanks to the faculty in Small Animal Internal Medicine, who provided clinical coverage during my sabbatical leave thereby providing me the time needed to focus on this endeavor. I am thankful for the staff at the UC Davis Veterinary Medical Teaching Hospital who ensured that my patients were evaluated safely, effectively, and efficiently. A special thank you to John Doval for his expert assistance in generating images for this book.

I am also exceptionally grateful to my colleagues at the University of Melbourne, Australia, who hosted my sabbatical leave. The generosity, enthusiasm, and encouragement that they offered were unsurpassed, and they provided me with the utmost support in all my academic and scholarly endeavors.

Clinical Canine and Feline
Respiratory Medicine

Localization of Disease

1

Clinical signs that provide clues to the existence of respiratory disease include nasal discharge, cough, respiratory noise, tachypnea, difficulty breathing, or exercise intolerance. The first step toward making a diagnosis requires accurate localization of the anatomic origin of disease within the respiratory tract: the nasal cavity, upper or lower airway, lung parenchyma, or pleural space. This will allow construction of an accurate list of differential diagnoses, will facilitate efficient diagnostic testing, and will allow rational empiric therapy while waiting for test results.

Nasal Discharge

History

Nasal discharge is almost always a sign of local disease within the nasal cavity. One exception is eosinophilic bronchopneumopathy, an inflammatory condition of the lung and airways that can also involve the nasal epithelium. A second exception can be found in the dog or cat with lower respiratory tract disease (usually bacterial pneumonia) that coughs airway material into the nasopharynx, which subsequently drains from the nose. In both situations, animals usually have a combination of cough and nasal discharge. The most common causes of nasal discharge include infectious, inflammatory, and neoplastic disorders as well as dental-related nasal disease and foreign bodies (Table 1.1). Additional clinical signs that can be seen in animals with nasal disease include sneezing or reverse sneezing, pawing or rubbing at the face, noisy breathing or mouth breathing, facial pain, or an unexplained odor near the head.

Table 1.1. Causes of nasal discharge in dogs and cats

	Dog	Cat
Infectious	Canine infectious respiratory disease complex[a]	Acute upper respiratory tract disease complex[b]
	Aspergillus	*Cryptococcus*
	Penicillium	*Aspergillus*
	Rhinosporidium	
Inflammatory	Lymphoplasmacytic rhinitis	Feline chronic rhinosinusitis
Neoplastic	Adenocarcinoma	Lymphoma
	Sarcomas	Adenocarcinoma
	Lymphoma	Sarcomas
Local	Tooth root abscess	Nasal or nasopharyngeal polyp
	Oronasal fistula	Tooth root abscess
	Trauma	Oronasal fistula
	Foreign body	Foreign body
	Nasal or nasopharyngeal polyp	Trauma
Other	Primary ciliary dyskinesia	Primary ciliary dyskinesia
	Nasal mites	
	Xeromycteria (dry nose syndrome)	

[a]Reported causes include canine adenovirus-2, canine parainfluenza-3 virus, canine respiratory coronavirus, canine herpesvirus, canine distemper virus, *Bordetella* and *Mycoplasma*. Canine influenza virus is a new addition to the list of etiologic agents.
[b]Reported causes include feline herpesvirus-1, feline calicivirus, *Chlamydophila*, *Bordetella*, and *Mycoplasma*.

When evaluating the animal with nasal discharge, important considerations include the duration of signs, the type of discharge as well as changes in its character over time, and the presence of unilateral or bilateral signs. Acute nasal discharge is often accompanied by sneezing and is most commonly associated with viral upper respiratory tract disease or a foreign body. Animals with acute nasal discharge usually have dramatic clinical signs that either resolve within a week without treatment or are so severe that animals are rapidly evaluated by a veterinarian. More frustrating cases are those with chronic nasal discharge, which often have low level but progressive signs from weeks to months to years before the severity of disease prompts veterinary care.

With many causes of nasal disease including viral disease or foreign body, discharge is serous initially and then progresses to a mucoid character when inflammation induces mucus production or when secondary bacterial infection develops. Yellow-green nasal discharge can be an indicator of eosinophilic disease but is also encountered in other inflammatory conditions, while brown-tinged discharge suggests the presence of blood within the mucus. Bright red blood can be found in combination with nasal discharge because of trauma to blood vessels associated with the primary disease process or due to the severity of sneezing. Pure epistaxis has been associated with local causes of disease, including inflammatory rhinitis, canine aspergillosis, and neoplasia; however, systemic vascular disorders must also be considered including coagulopathies and systemic hypertension.

Nasal discharge that is strictly unilateral is most suspicious for local disease due to a foreign body, trauma, tooth root abscess or oronasal fistula, or an early fungal infection or neoplasm. However, systemic vascular disease or a coagulopathy can result in unilateral signs. Also, inflammatory diseases such as lymphoplasmacytic rhinitis in the dog and feline chronic rhinosinusitis can also present with lateralizing clinical signs, although in most cases, imaging and histology reveal that both sides of the nasal cavity are affected.

Signalment

Young animals with nasal discharge are most often affected by infectious upper respiratory tract diseases. A nasopharyngeal polyp should be considered when discharge is accompanied by obstructed breathing. Primary ciliary dyskinesia is a defect of innate immunity that results in effectual mucociliary clearance, failure to clear secretions, and recurrent infection. Therefore, this condition would be more frequently recognized in a younger animal. Affected dogs are often purebred, with an increased prevalence in the Bichon Frise, although any breed of dog or cat can be affected. While neoplastic disease most typically affects older animals, it also occurs in animals 2–4 years of age and can be particularly aggressive, especially in dogs. Canine aspergillosis is most often encountered in younger dogs and older cats. Cryptococcus and inflammatory rhinitis can affect dogs or cats of any age.

Nasal disease of most types (fungal, neoplastic, and inflammatory) is most commonly found in dolicocephalic dog breeds. An unusual combination of rhinitis and bronchopneumonia has been reported in the Irish wolfhound, where a genetic defect in respiratory immunity is suspected.

Physical Examination

A complete physical examination is essential in every animal presented for evaluation of respiratory disease. In animals with nasal discharge, important features to focus on include the presence or absence of nasal airflow, changes in ocular retropulsion, lack of soft palate depression, regional local lymph node enlargement, and facial asymmetry or pain. These parts of the physical examination are most important because they can help identify the space-occupying nature of some nasal diseases, particularly nasal neoplasia, feline cryptococcosis, and nasopharyngeal polyps, and because these findings can detect local extension or metastasis.

Nasal airflow can be assessed by holding a chilled microscope in front of each nostril to show fogging of the glass or by using a wisp of cotton (from a cotton ball or Q-tip) to watch for air movement. The mouth should be held closed during the procedure, and occlusion of the alternate nostril can be helpful for enhancing airflow through the side of the nasal cavity to be examined (Figure 1.1). An animal with a mass effect in the nasal cavity or nasopharynx will fail to fog the glass or move the cotton wisp and will often object to this manipulation because it obstructs airflow. Conversely, even animals with heavy mucus accumulation in the nasal cavity will retain nasal airflow.

Facial palpation is performed to assess for a pain response, to locate swellings and depressions in bony structures, and to check for symmetry of the skull. Ocular retropulsion is a part of the facial examination and is performed by placing each thumb over the closed lids and pressing gently backward, upward, medially, and laterally (Figure 1.2). Nasal lesions that are producing a mass effect behind the globe (primarily a neoplasm

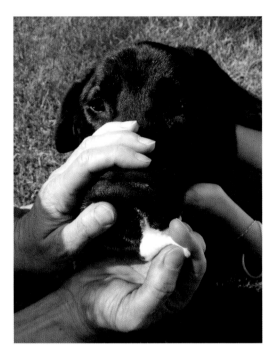

Figure 1.1. Nasal airflow can be assessed by occluding one nostril and assessing flow from the alternate nostril with a cotton wisp or chilled microscope slide.

or retrobulbar abscess) will cause a lateralizing difference in the resistance to depression. Similarly, palpation within the oral cavity can reveal bony abnormalities in the hard palate or might suggest a mass lesion above the soft palate. To perform this examination, the mouth is held open, and the roof of the mouth is palpated from the front of the hard

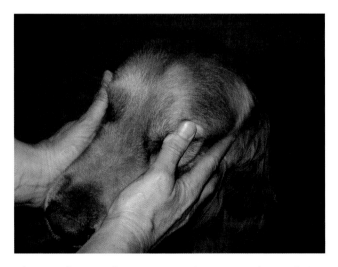

Figure 1.2. Palpation during ocular retropulsion can suggest the presence of a mass lesion within the optic tract.

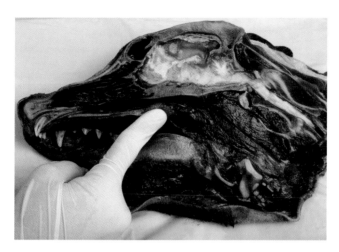

Figure 1.3.   In the normal animal, palpation of the soft palate will readily depress tissue into the nasopharyngeal region. The presence of a mass lesion in the nasopharynx will result in resistance to depression.

palate through to the end of the soft palate. In the normal animal, the soft palate is readily depressed upward into the nasopharyngeal region (Figure 1.3). A mass in this area (most commonly a neoplasm, fungal granuloma, or polyp) will resist depression. The dental arcade should also be evaluated during the oral examination, although it is important to remember that tooth root disease can be present in the absence of external signs.

Neoplastic disease, fungal infection, or inflammatory diseases within the nasal cavity can involve mandibular lymph nodes and the disease process can sometimes be identified by cytology of a lymph node aspirate, even when there is no palpable enlargement. Nasal depigmentation is a relatively specific feature of canine nasal aspergillosis found in up to 40% of cases and is thought to result from elaboration of a dermonecrotic toxin by the fungus.

Loud Breathing

Definition

Loud breathing most commonly results from a disorder affecting the nasal cavity or upper airway (larynx, pharynx, or cervical trachea), although occasionally animals with lower airway disease will present for loud breathing. Stertor is a gurgling or snoring sound that is produced as air flows past a soft tissue obstruction. It can be caused by narrowing of the nasal cavity, by elongation or thickening of the soft palate, or by edema or eversion of laryngeal saccules. It varies in tone and pitch, and it may be audible on both inspiration and expiration. In contrast, stridor is classically an inspiratory noise of a single, high pitch that results from rapid flow of air past a rigid obstruction, such as a paralyzed or collapsed larynx. Stridor can also be heard in an animal with a laryngeal mass effect, or occasionally in an animal with nasopharyngeal stenosis or fixed cervical tracheal collapse or stenosis.

Signalment

Stertor is commonly encountered in brachycephalic dog breeds such as bulldogs (English and French), Pugs, and Boston Terriers and is also seen in Himalayan and Persian cats. Loud breathing is often present early in life and becomes worse with development of additional respiratory disease or with weight gain. Some animals are not presented for evaluation of stertor and respiratory difficulty until late in life because of the perception that noisy respiration is "normal" for the breed.

Animals with stridor due to congenital laryngeal paralysis are usually young (6–12 weeks) when the disease is manifest. Affected breeds include the Dalmatian, Rottweiler, Great Pyrenees, Bouvier des Flandres, Siberian Husky, White German Shepherd, and some cats (see Chapter 5). Acquired laryngeal paralysis is most commonly found in older large breed dogs such as Labrador and Golden retrievers. Brachycephalic breed dogs that develop laryngeal collapse are usually older at the time of diagnosis, however because this is an end-stage manifestation of airway obstruction, age varies depending on the severity of disease.

Physical Examination

In a normal animal, breathing is quiet at rest. Stertor and stridor can be heard without the use of a stethoscope; however, in some instances, careful auscultation over the neck region is needed to confirm stridor. Increasing respiratory flow rate by gentle exercise can improve detection of stridor; however, panting must be discouraged. In the normal animal, auscultation over the larynx and trachea will reveal loud, hollow sounds that are heard equally on inspiration and expiration. Because upper respiratory noises are typically loud and can obscure lung sounds, auscultation of the larynx and tracheal region is recommended in all patients/prior to thoracic auscultation to improve differentiation of upper from lower respiratory sounds and to improve detection of heart sounds. This is particularly helpful in brachycephalic breeds (Figure 1.4). Brachycephalic breeds commonly have visible stenotic nares as part of the disease complex, and excessive oropharyngeal folds may be evident.

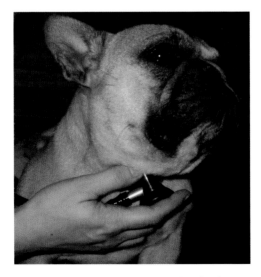

Figure 1.4. Prior to thoracic auscultation, the laryngeal and cervical tracheal regions are ausculted to define upper airway sounds.

Cough

History

Cough occurs because of activation of irritant receptors that lie between epithelial cells lining the airways and can be triggered by inflammatory products of neutrophils or eosinophils, by the presence of excess secretions, and by airway compression or collapse (Table 1.2). Important historical features to determine include the onset and duration of cough, the character of the cough, and environmental features that appear to trigger cough.

Animals with a wet- or moist-sounding cough most likely have excessive airway secretions due to infectious or inflammatory airway or parenchymal disease. Observant owners of the animal with a productive cough may note that the animal swallows after coughing or retches to remove secretions from the airway. However, infectious, inflammatory, and structural diseases of the airway can also result in a dry cough when secretions are minimal or early in the course of disease. Cough in animals with airway disease is often harsh and can be chronic, intermittent, or paroxysmal in nature. Animals with pneumonia may have a softer cough along with a vague history of illness characterized by anorexia and lethargy.

Determining environmental and travel history is important for animals with cough. Exposure to a high-density dog population should raise concern for disease associated with canine respiratory disease complex. If the cough is harsh and dry, *Bordetella* should be considered, while a soft, chronic cough could be suggestive of canine influenza virus infection. Sporting dogs that develop an acute onset of cough or have a chronic, antibiotic-responsive cough may have foreign body pneumonia. Fungal pneumonia should be suspected in animals with cough that have traveled to endemic regions. In those animals, cough is usually

Table 1.2.   Respiratory causes of cough in dogs and cats

	Dog	Cat
Infectious tracheobronchitis	Canine infectious respiratory disease complex[a]	*Mycoplasma* *Bordetella*
Pneumonia	Bacterial Aspiration Foreign body Fungal Eosinophilic Interstitial	Bacterial Aspiration Foreign body Fungal Interstitial
Inflammation	Chronic bronchitis Eosinophilic bronchopneumopathy	Asthma/chronic bronchitis
Neoplasia	Primary Metastatic	Primary Metastatic
Structural	Bronchiectasis Airway collapse	Bronchiectasis

[a]Reported causes include canine adenovirus-2, canine parainfluenza-3 virus, canine respiratory coronavirus, canine herpesvirus and canine distemper virus along with *Bordetella* and *Mycoplasma*. Canine influenza virus can also be included in the list of etiologic agents.

accompanied by tachypnea and systemic signs of illness. Finally, environmental history is important because exposure to pollutants and airway irritants can exacerbate upper or lower airway diseases in both dogs and cats.

Physical Examination

One of the more difficult challenges in assessing animals with respiratory disease is the development of good auscultation skills. Practice and patience are required because audible sounds are altered by age, body condition score, conformation, respiratory pattern, and the presence of disease. As mentioned earlier, careful examination should include the larynx and trachea, followed by auscultation of all lung fields. The anatomic origin for lung sounds has not been fully established; however, normal lung sounds are usually designated as bronchial, vesicular, or bronchovesicular. Bronchial sounds are loud and are heard best over the large airways near the hilus. Typically, they are louder and longer during expiration than inspiration and have a tubular character. Vesicular lung sounds are soft, heard best on inspiration, and can be detected over the periphery of the chest in normal animals. The sound resembles a breeze passing through leaves on a tree. Bronchovesicular sounds (a mixture of bronchial and vesicular qualities) can be heard on inspiration more than expiration.

Lung sounds in animals with airway or parenchymal disease are often increased in loudness or harshness. Adventitious (abnormal) lung sounds (crackles and wheezes) are discontinuous noises that should always be taken as an indicator of disease. Crackles are thought to result from rapid opening of airways but could also arise from equalization in pressure as air passes through fluid or mucus-filled airways. They can be heard at any point during inspiration or expiration. Wheezes result from air passing through airways narrowed by intraluminal mucus, extraluminal compression, or by collapse or constriction, and are usually heard on expiration. Adventitious lung sounds can be enhanced by inducing a cough or a deep breath, or by exercising the patient. In normal animals, it is difficult to induce a cough by palpating the trachea; however, animals with airway or parenchymal disease usually have increased tracheal sensitivity due to activation of irritant receptors by infection or inflammation.

Fine crackles are suggestive of pulmonary edema, particularly if ausculted in the hilar region of a dog, whereas coarse crackles are more suggestive of pneumonia or airway disease. Dogs or cats with pulmonary fibrosis can display either fine or coarse crackles that are auscultable diffusely across the chest. Auscultation in dogs with airway collapse can reveal diffuse crackling sounds because of the presence of concurrent bronchitis or because of small airways that suddenly pop open. A loud snapping sound over the hilar region at end expiration is suggestive of collapse of the intrathoracic trachea, carina, or mainstem bronchi.

Tachypnea

History

Tachypnea is most often associated with parenchymal or pleural disease, although in the cat, tachypnea can also be seen with bronchial disease. Therefore, in the cat, tachypnea can be found in conjunction with historical features of cough and decreased activity. Parenchymal diseases that lead to tachypnea are primarily pneumonia and pulmonary edema, and these disorders can be acute or chronic and insidious in onset. They are typically associated with systemic signs of illness such as lethargy, anorexia, and weight loss. Tachypnea due to with pneumothorax is usually acute; however, pleural effusive disorders can result in either an acute presentation with respiratory distress or a more chronic development of signs due to slow accumulation of fluid. Usually, the degree of respiratory distress is associated with the rapidity of fluid or air accumulation rather than with the specific volume present. Cats seem to be particularly sensitive to addition of a final, critical volume of fluid that overcomes their ability to compensate for filling of the pleural space.

Physical Examination

Cervical and thoracic auscultation as described for evaluation of animals with cough is important for animals that present with tachypnea since many diseases will result in both clinical signs. In addition to listening for increased sounds, it is important to determine if there is an absence of lung sounds, which might indicate either lung consolidation or the presence of fluid or air in the pleural space.

A notable clinical sign associated with parenchymal or pleural disease is a rapid, shallow breathing pattern, although with pleural disease, exaggerated chest wall motion can sometimes be present. In animals with severe respiratory distress, elbows are abducted and the neck is extended to facilitate movement of air into the alveoli. Parenchymal diseases are characterized by increased lung sounds or detection of adventitious sounds. When pleural effusion is present, lung sounds are ausculted in the dorsal fields only and muffled sounds are heard ventrally; heart sounds are also muffled. Pneumothorax leads to an absence of lung sounds dorsally due to compression by air, and lung sounds are present in the ventral fields only.

In addition to auscultation, thoracic percussion aids in determining if pleural disease is present. Percussion can be performed using a pleximeter and mallet or by placing the fingers of one hand on the chest and rapidly striking them with fingers of the opposite hand (Figure 1.5). The sound that develops varies depending on whether an air or fluid density is

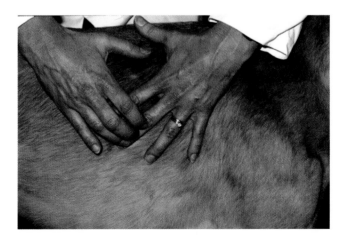

Figure 1.5. Each region of the thorax should be percussed to detect regional differences in the air/soft tissue sounds that are created. One hand is placed against the thorax and is rapped quickly and sharply with the curved fingers of the alternate hand.

present within the thoracic cage. Percussion of the chest in a region filled with fluid reveals a dull sound while in an animal with pneumothorax or air trapping, percussion results in increased resonance. This technique is somewhat limited in a cat or small dog because of the small size of the thoracic cavity.

Careful auscultation of the heart is also indicated in animals with parenchymal or pleural disease because congestive heart failure can lead to respiratory signs due to pulmonary edema or pleural effusion. In such a case, a heart murmur or gallop would be expected along with tachycardia, and jugular veins are often distended in an animal with right ventricular failure. If the apical impulse is poorly audible, this is an additional clue to the presence of pleural effusion.

Exercise Intolerance

History

In general, exercise intolerance can result from respiratory, cardiac, musculoskeletal, neurologic, or metabolic diseases. Respiratory disorders that result in exercise intolerance usually do so through airway obstruction in diseases such as laryngeal paralysis or bronchitis, or through hypoxemia associated with parenchymal disease. Historical features in animals with airway obstruction can include loud breathing noises as well as progressive tiring and a reduced level of activity. Upper airway obstruction due to laryngeal disease may be accompanied by reports of dysphonia, decreased vocalization, gagging, or retching, while lower airway obstruction due to bronchoconstriction or inflammation is usually associated with cough.

Physical Examination

In the older, large breed dog presented for evaluation of exercise intolerance, careful attention should be paid to laryngeal auscultation for stridor suggestive of laryngeal paralysis. Increased tracheal sensitivity and loud or adventitious lung sounds in cats or dogs with exercise intolerance but no systemic signs of illness suggest that bronchial narrowing or inflammation may be responsible for exercise intolerance. Animals that display tachypnea on physical examination, abnormal lung sounds, and systemic signs of illness likely suffer from some form of pneumonia.

Respiratory Diagnostics 2

General

Laboratory Testing

Basic blood work (complete blood count and biochemical panel) are often performed during the workup of a respiratory patient and may help support the presence of an underlying respiratory tract disease. In local diseases associated with inflammation or infection such as rhinitis and tracheobronchitis, hematologic changes are rarely found. With parenchymal diseases such as bacterial or aspiration pneumonia, a neutrophilic leukocytosis is often found. Neutrophilia or eosinophilia is reported in eosinophilic pneumonia/bronchopneumopathy and feline bronchial disease. Fungal pneumonia is anticipated to result in neutrophilia and monocytosis, reflecting the chronic nature of disease. Chronic hypoxemia can result in polycythemia.

Biochemical abnormalities in respiratory diseases are usually nonspecific. Hyperglobulinemia can be found in feline bronchial disease, fungal pneumonia, chronic foreign body or aspiration pneumonia, or bronchiectasis due to chronic antigenic stimulation, and concurrent hypoalbuminemia is occasionally present as a negative acute phase reactant.

Molecular diagnostics are increasingly used to document the presence of an infectious organism, such as feline herpesvirus-1, *Bordetella*, or *Mycoplasma*, in either upper or lower respiratory tract disease; however, there are important limitations to interpretation of results (see sections on specific diseases). Also, it is critical to realize that a positive molecular assay does not confirm that the organism is responsible for the clinical disease identified.

Pulse Oximetry

Pulse oximetry provides an estimate of hemoglobin saturation with oxygen and is inexpensive, noninvasive, and easy to perform. The technique relies on detection of the optical density of the pulse wave as blood passes through the arterial system. The sensor subtracts the signal between pulses from the height of the pulse wave to determine oxygenation of inflowing blood only. Because of this feature, pulse oximetry can provide a falsely low measurement in a hypotensive patient with weak pulses or in an animal with anemia. This technique cannot differentiate between methemoglobin and oxyhemoglobin.

Pulse oximetry is useful prior to anesthetizing the patient for a respiratory procedure or as a monitoring tool during therapy. Sites that can used to obtain a measurement include the lip, tongue, between the toes, on the ear pinna, and sometimes on the abdomen. The probe can be applied to various sites several times to obtain a signal, and detection of a strong pulse rate indicates that the reading is likely accurate. A pulse oximeter reading below 95% correlates with a P_aO_2 of less than 80 mm Hg (Figure 2.1). When such a reading is obtained, an arterial blood gas analysis should be performed, if available, to confirm the degree of hypoxemia. It is important to remember that the pulse oximeter measures only oxygenation. It provides no information on ventilatory status and thus cannot detect hypoventilation (increased P_aCO_2) in an animal.

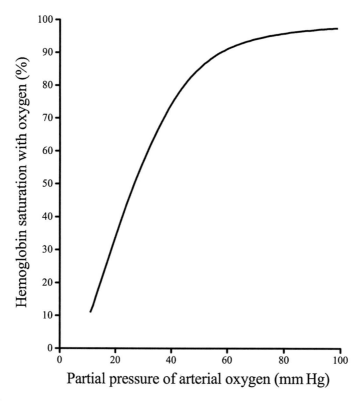

Figure 2.1. Pulse oximetry measures hemoglobin saturation with oxygen, which has a sigmoidal relationship with the partial pressure of arterial oxygen. A hemoglobin saturation <95% equates to a P_aO_2 <80 mm Hg and indicates hypoxemia.

Pulse oximetry can be valuable in determining response to therapy in hypoxemic patients because improvements in oxygenation occur prior to radiographic changes. However, because of the sigmoidal relationship between hemoglobin saturation and arterial oxygen, oximetry remains a somewhat crude estimate of lung function.

Arterial Blood Gas Analysis

Arterial samples are obtained by direct puncture of the dorsal metatarsal artery in dogs and the femoral artery in cats and small dogs. A small needle (23–25 gauge) on a heparinized syringe is used, or a self-filling syringe can be used. The artery is palpated and stabilized with two fingers of one hand while the syringe is firmly placed through the wall of the artery. Approximately 0.5-mL blood is needed for analysis and the sample must be stoppered and stored on ice until analyzed. After withdrawal of the syringe, firm pressure is applied to the artery for 3–5 minutes. An arterial blood gas analysis measures P_aO_2, P_aCO_2, pH, total CO_2, and hemoglobin saturation with oxygen, and allows calculation of bicarbonate, base excess and deficit, and oxygen content (Table 2.1).

Alveolar–arterial oxygen gradient and PF ratio

The alveolar–arterial (A–a) oxygen gradient estimates the difference between the calculated alveolar oxygen level expected for the animal and the measured arterial oxygen level. Thus, the A–a gradient corrects for the level of ventilation performed by the animal and allows comparison of blood gas data through the course of disease that is not impacted by the effect of an increase or a decrease in P_aCO_2 on P_aO_2. The A–a oxygen gradient is calculated as

$$A-a = F_iO_2(PB - PH_2O) - (P_aCO_2 \div 0.9) - P_aO_2$$

where F_iO_2 is the fraction of inspired oxygen (0.21 on room air), PB is the barometric pressure (in mm Hg), PH_2O is the water vapor pressure (47 mm Hg at 37°C), and R is the respiratory quotient (ratio of CO_2 production to O_2 consumption, usually assigned a value between 0.8 and 1.0). P_aO_2 and P_aCO_2 are obtained from blood gas analysis. Normal value is <15.

The PaO_2/FiO_2 ratio (PF or oxygenation ratio) provides a measure of the ability of the lung to oxygenate as the fraction of inspired oxygen changes from room air to 100% oxygen. This is calculated by dividing arterial oxygen by FiO_2 (ranging from 0.21 to 1.0). Normal animals have a PF ratio of >500. Values between 300 and 500 indicate mild impairment

Table 2.1. Normal blood gas values for dogs and cats

	Dog	Cat
PaO_2 (mm Hg)	90 (80–105)	100 (95–105)
$PaCO_2$ (mm Hg)	37 (32–43)	31 (26–36)
pH	7.35–7.45	7.35–7.45
HCO_3 (mmol/L)	22 (18–26)	18 (14–22)

Table 2.2. Respiratory causes of hypoxemia

Mechanism	Clinical Attributes	Causes
Hypoventilation	High P_aCO_2 Normal A–a gradient Improved by oxygen supplementation Improved by increasing alveolar ventilation	Anesthesia Upper airway obstruction Neuromuscular weakness CNS disease
V/Q mismatch	Increased A–a gradient Mildly increased P_aCO_2 Markedly improved by oxygen supplementation	Virtually any lung disease
Shunt	Increased A–a gradient Not improved by oxygen supplementation Not improved by increasing alveolar ventilation	Congenital right to left cardiac shunts Acute respiratory distress syndrome
Diffusion impairment	Increased A–a gradient Seldom a major cause of hypoxemia at rest Causes hypoxemia during exercise or with low inspired oxygen Improved by oxygen supplementation	Interstitial lung disease Pulmonary edema
Reduced inspired oxygen	Improved by oxygen Causes hypoxemia during exercise or when diffusion is impaired	High altitude

of oxygenation, while values <200 indicate serious decrements in oxygenation. A PF ratio <200 is one of the requirements for a diagnosis of acute respiratory distress syndrome.

Causes of hypoxemia

Obtaining an arterial blood gas, calculating the A–a gradient, and assessing response of hemoglobin saturation or P_aO_2 to exogenous oxygen supplementation allow assumptions to be made about the most likely mechanism causing hypoxemia (Table 2.2). This can help determine the most likely underlying cause of hypoxemia, although ventilation/perfusion mismatch contributes to the pathophysiology of hypoxemia in almost all lung diseases.

Imaging

Radiography is often the key to creating an appropriate list of differential diagnoses for the respiratory case and for determining the type of sampling method that is most likely to achieve a final diagnosis, such as endoscopy, fine-needle aspiration (FNA), or a tracheal wash (Table 2.3). It will also help determine the need for advanced imaging including fluoroscopy, ultrasound, nuclear scintigraphy, or computed tomography. Specific features of these tests are presented in the relevant disease sections.

Table 2.3.　Airway-sampling techniques for various lung patterns

Radiographic Pattern	Differential Diagnoses	Sampling Technique
Interstitial	Viral pneumonia Rickettsial pneumonia Protozoal pneumonia Hemorrhage Vasculitis Pulmonary fibrosis Neoplasia Early pulmonary edema Aspiration pneumonia	Fine-needle aspirate Lung biopsy Bronchoscopy Tracheal wash
Bronchial	Chronic bronchitis Feline bronchitis/asthma Bronchiectasis Parasitic bronchitis Early bronchopneumonia	Tracheal wash Bronchoscopy
Alveolar	Bronchopneumonia Aspiration pneumonia Fungal pneumonia Hemorrhage Pulmonary edema Neoplasia Noncardiogenic pulmonary edema	Tracheal wash Bronchoscopy
Consolidation	Neoplasia Lung lobe torsion Consolidating pneumonia Granuloma Bronchial obstruction Feline bronchitis Foreign body inhalation	Bronchoscopy Fine-needle aspirate Tracheal wash
Vascular	Congenital heart disease Congestive heart failure Heartworm disease Pulmonary hypertension Pulmonary thromboembolism	Echocardiography
Effusion	Hydrothorax Pyothorax Hemothorax Chylothorax Neoplasia Diaphragmatic hernia	Thoracocentesis

Airway Sampling

Transoral Tracheal Wash

Transoral tracheal wash is appropriate for use in large and small dogs or in cats. A sterile endotracheal tube and a sterile polypropylene or blunt-ended red rubber catheter (3.5–8 French) are needed. Prior to doing a tracheal wash, the catheter should be measured against the animal and marked at a position that estimates the location of the carina, which is approximately at the fourth intercostal space. Passing the catheter too far distally can result in airway damage. The animal is anesthetized with a short-acting anesthetic agent. Options include propofol, ketamine–valium, or a balanced protocol using a narcotic agent. Prior to intubation, the function of the larynx is assessed. In the cat, local lidocaine can be used to facilitate intubation and avoid contamination of the tube through contact with oropharyngeal or laryngeal mucosa. An assistant holds the tube in place during the lavage; however, if retrieval of fluid is less than desired, the cuff of the endotracheal tube can be inflated to improve suction.

With the endotracheal tube held in place, the polypropylene or red rubber catheter is passed sterilely to the level of the carina, and the three-way stopcock with syringe is attached to the outer port. An aliquot of saline (4–6 mL) is instilled into the airway, and suction is used to retrieve the fluid and cells from the lower airway. Either hand suction or house suction can be applied as needed. Retrieval of fluid can be enhanced by having the assistant compress the chest or by stimulating a cough during suction. Instillation and aspiration of fluid can be repeated several times until an adequate sample has been retrieved (0.5–1.0 mL is usually sufficient for culture and cytology).

A modification of the transoral tracheal wash can be performed, which yields a sample more closely approximating that of a bronchoalveolar lavage. In the dog, this is achieved using a 16-French Argyle™ stomach tube (Sherwood Medical Co/Tyco Healthcare Kendall, Deland, FL) (Hawkins and Berry 1999). The dog must be large enough to accommodate an endotracheal tube that will not be fully occluded by the stomach tube. The stomach tube is shortened to remove any side holes on the distal end of the tube and to create a length that approximates the distance from the endotracheal tube to the last rib. The distal end of the tube can be tapered with a pencil sharpener to improve the ability to wedge within the airway, and the tube should be sterilized prior to use. Endotracheal intubation is carried out using a short-acting anesthetic agent (e.g., propofol) and a sterile endotracheal tube. The dog is placed in dorsal recumbency, and the modified stomach tube is passed through the lumen of the endotracheal tube until it meets resistance. Gentle pressure should be used when passing and wedging this tube to avoid perforating the lung. As soon as slight resistance is encountered, the tube is withdrawn 1–2 cm and lavage is initiated with 20 mL of sterile saline followed by 5 mL of air. Gentle hand suction is applied to retrieve the fluid, and a second aliquot can be instilled as needed.

Nonbronchoscopic bronchoalveolar lavage (BAL) has also been reported in the cat, and the cell distribution obtained on cytology matches that found with bronchoscopy (Hawkins et al. 1994). For this procedure, the cat is anesthetized with a short-acting anesthetic agent (ketamine–valium in a 1:1 mixture or propofol) and intubated with a sterile endotracheal tube. The cuff is inflated and the cat is placed in lateral recumbency with the most affected side down. Aliquots (1–3 as needed) of warmed sterile 0.9% saline (5 ml/kg) are instilled directly into the endotracheal tube using a 35-mL syringe with syringe adapter. Fluid is retrieved by hand aspiration. Elevating the hindquarters can facilitate collection, and approximately 65–70% fluid retrieval should be expected. Alternately, a dog urinary catheter (6–8 French) can be passed gently through a sterile endotracheal tube until resistance is met, in a manner similar to that employed when a modified stomach tube is used to perform blind BAL in a dog (Foster et al. 2004). Instillation of 5–10 mL of sterile saline provides an adequate lavage sample for cultures and cytology. With either procedure, respiratory rate and pulse oximetry should be monitored to detect untoward reactions and oxygen supplied as needed.

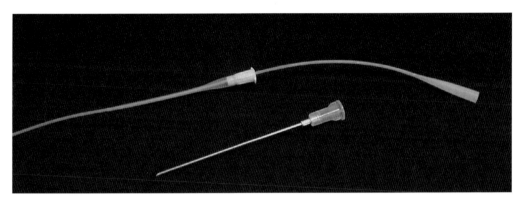

Figure 2.2.   An over-the-needle catheter can be used as a cannula to perform a tracheal wash using a sterile urinary catheter.

Transtracheal Wash

Transtracheal wash is appropriate for larger dogs (>8 kg) or those that cannot be anesthetized for a transoral tracheal wash. Generally only local anesthesia is needed although a mild sedative may facilitate completion of the procedure. The easiest way to perform a transtracheal wash is with a through-the-needle jugular catheter. An alternate approach is to use a 16-gauge over-the-needle catheter as a cannula to penetrate the trachea and a long, sterile 3.5-French urinary catheter to pass down into the airways for sample collection (Figure 2.2). The trachea can be entered at the cricothyroid notch but is preferable to enter the trachea between the tracheal rings lower on the neck to avoid potential damage to laryngeal structures. This will also facilitate collection of a sample from more distal airways since the jugular catheter is relatively short in length. For either technique, the ventral portion of the neck is clipped and lightly scrubbed with antiseptic solution followed by alcohol wipes. A more complete surgical preparation is performed after local anesthesia is instilled.

Local anesthesia with lidocaine (0.25–0.5 mL) is used at two sites that will be penetrated by the needle: at the skin and between the tracheal rings. The needle of the jugular catheter will penetrate the skin low on the neck, and the skin will then be drawn upward prior to entering the airway lumen. This creates a subcutaneous seal that limits air leakage between the skin entry and the airway.

To begin catheter placement, the needle is placed into the trachea with the bevel of the needle facing downward so that the catheter will pass over the short edge of needle rather than the long edge as it is advanced through the lumen. This makes it less likely that the sharp edge of the needle will cut off the catheter during passage. Tent the skin and pass the needle or catheter through the site that has been infiltrated with lidocaine. The needle or catheter is directed perpendicular to the trachea initially (Figure 2.3). When preparing to enter between the tracheal rings, stabilize the trachea firmly against the neck to prevent it from moving away from needle. After the needle has passed through the skin and subcutaneous tissue, the skin is retracted upward to enter the airway one to two tracheal rings above the site where the skin was penetrated. A distinct pop is usually felt when the needle enters the tracheal lumen, and the dog often coughs. With the needle in the airway, the angle made between the catheter and trachea is decreased to 60° to facilitate passage of the catheter down the

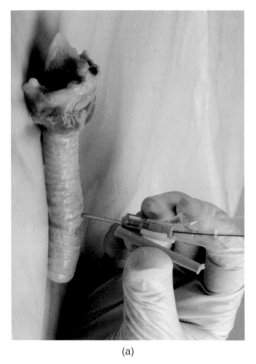
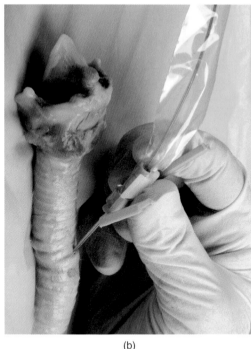

(a)　　　　　　　　　　　　　　　　　　　(b)

Figure 2.3. To initiate a tracheal wash, the needle is directed into the trachea at a perpendicular angle (a). After the needle has penetrated between the tracheal rings, the hub of the needle (or the catheter being used as the cannula) is moved toward the neck to create a more parallel angle for passage of the long catheter down the trachea (b).

lumen of the airway (Figure 2.3). The needle is withdrawn at this stage to pass the sampling catheter through the short catheter to the level of the carina (Figure 2.4).

When using the jugular catheter system, after the catheter is passed partially down the trachea, the needle is withdrawn from the neck (taking care that the catheter does not also come out), and the needle guard is secured in place before any manipulations of the system are made to decrease the risk of shearing off the catheter with the needle.

The tracheal wash catheter should move freely down the airway and passage usually stimulates coughing. If this does not result in a cough, the catheter may be traveling in subcutaneous tissue and it should be removed. If this occurs when using the jugular catheter system, the needle and catheter should be withdrawn together, without retracting the catheter back into the needle to avoid shearing off the catheter in the airway.

When the catheter is fully deployed, the stylet is withdrawn to perform the transtracheal wash. An aliquot of saline (4–10 mL) is instilled into the airway, and suction is used to retrieve the fluid and cells from the lower airway.

Respiratory Endoscopy

Rhinoscopy

A full rhinoscopic examination includes evaluation of the caudal nasopharynx to visualize the opening at the choanae and inspection of the rostral nasal cavity. The best equipment

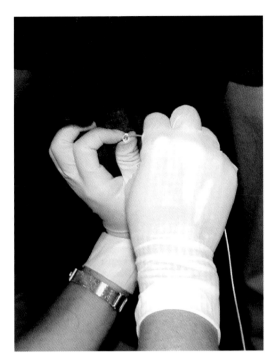

Figure 2.4.   The cannula catheter has been seated between the tracheal rings and the long catheter is being passed down the trachea for collection of an airway sample.

to use in evaluating the caudal nasopharynx is a flexible endoscope. If this is unavailable, a bright light source and dental mirror can be used, along with a spay hook to retract the soft palate cranially. Examining the nasopharynx is a highly stimulatory procedure. Local anesthesia of the oropharynx with lidocaine gel can facilitate placement of the scope or the spay hook around the soft palate. Extending the neck and pulling the tongue forward will also help place the instruments in the proper position. The nonflexed scope is placed in the oral cavity and then flexed until the light can be seen above the soft palate (Figure 2.5). The scope is then pulled forward (with the flex in place) until the choanae is visualized. Note that the image is upside down and backward (Figure 2.6). Alternately, a dental mirror is placed in the back of the pharynx and angled above the soft palate while a light source is used to visualize the choanae. In some cases, rostral traction on the soft palate will facilitate visualization.

After the caudal nasopharynx is examined and samples are obtained for histopathology as indicated, a moistened lap pad is used to pack the throat and prevent aspiration during rostral rhinoscopy. Equipment available for rostral rhinoscopy includes rigid endoscopes (with or without an external sheath), otoscopes, and small fiberoptic endoscopes. Rigid scopes have better optics, are easier to maneuver, and come in smaller sizes while flexible scopes allow greater access to the nasal cavity and can permit examination of the frontal sinuses if there is marked turbinate destruction (such as in nasal aspergillosis). Rigid scopes are available with viewing angles of 0–30°. Rhinoscopy can be performed using the telescope portion of the rigid scope alone (~2.8 mm outer diameter) or by using the sheathed scope (~5 mm outer diameter), which has flush and suction ports as well as a biopsy port available

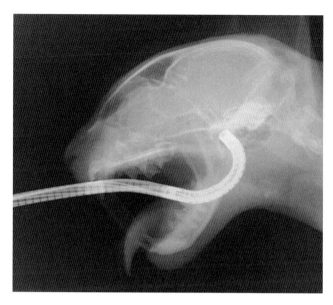

Figure 2.5. Visualization of the choanae is obtained by inserting a flexible endoscope into the oral cavity and flexing the scope maximally (180°) around the soft palate.

(Figure 2.7). The biopsy port of the sheath will accept standard endoscopic biopsy or foreign body retrieval instruments.

Before entering the nasal cavity, the endoscope is placed against the skull and measured to the level of the medial canthus of the eye to approximate the position of the cribriform plate. A piece of tape is applied to the instrument at this length, and the equipment should not be passed further than this point to avoid penetrating through the cribriform plate.

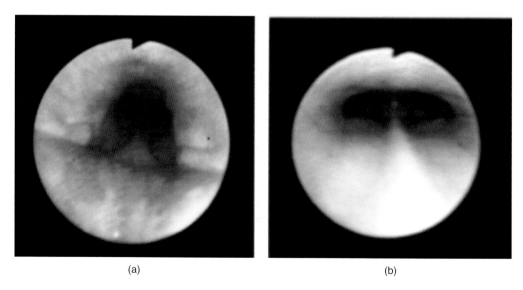

(a)   (b)

Figure 2.6. Image of the normal nasopharynx in a dog (a) and a cat (b).

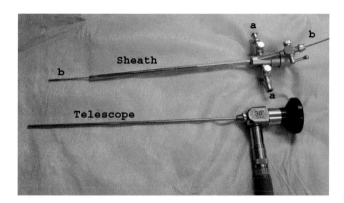

Figure 2.7. The sheath (~5-mm outer diameter) for the telescope portion of the rigid scope (~2.8-mm outer diameter) has flush and suction ports (a) as well as a biopsy port (b) available.

The normal nasal cavity is made up of scrolls of turbinates comprising the dorsal, middle, and ventral concha. The mucosa is generally pink with a pale sheen of serous secretion coating the smooth epithelial surface (Figure 2.8). The primary changes to look for are mucosal hyperemia, mucus accumulation, epithelial irregularities, turbinate destruction that is visualized as increased space between turbinates, and a mass effect that reduces space in the nasal cavity. When the cribriform plate is intact, nasal drops can be placed to achieve vasoconstriction (with oxymetazoline or phenylephrine) and/or topical anesthesia with tetracaine. This will cause swollen and hyperemic mucosa to blanch and shrink, thus changing the overall appearance of the mucosa but allowing improved access in some situations.

Mass lesions, fungal plaques, and specific mucosal lesions should be biopsied with visualization to improve the probability of achieving a diagnostic sample. With diffuse or generalized disease, an attempt should also be made to obtain at least the initial nasal

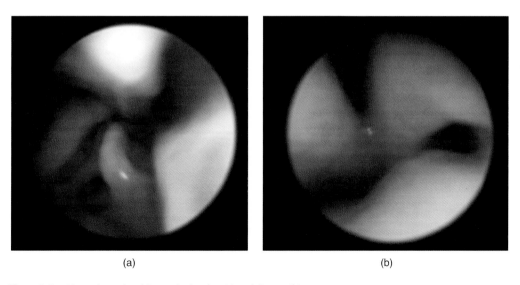

(a)   (b)

Figure 2.8. Normal nasal turbinates in the dog (a) and the cat (b).

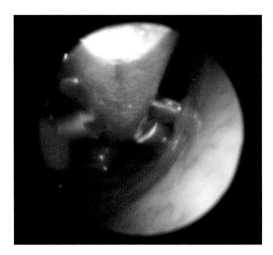

Figure 2.9. Diagnostic yield of a nasal biopsy sample is improved when the site to be sampled is visualized during the biopsy procedure.

biopsy with visualization of the area (Figure 2.9). This can be accomplished by using either the biopsy instrument that fits over the scope, by using a biopsy instrument that passes through the sheathed scope, or by advancing the biopsy instrument along the rigid scope. Once bleeding starts, the visual field is usually lost, although continuous or intermittent flush and suction can be used to clear the field. Nasal flush can be achieved by attaching a bag of chilled fluids to the port on the sheath of the scope or by inserting a red rubber catheter into the nasal cavity and using syringes to obtain a pulsatile pressurized flush. In cats, a 20–60-mL syringe inserted into the naris can be used for nasal flush (Figure 2.10). Nasal flush should also be used if excessive mucus obscures visualization of the nasal cavity. If a foreign body is highly suspected but is not visualized or removed during the procedure, nasal flush may dislodge the material. The soaked lap pad protecting the endotracheal tube should be removed, examined for foreign material periodically, and replaced with a new one. Also, if a foreign body is suspected, consider placing a Foley catheter in the caudal nasopharynx and using retrograde flush of the nasal cavities to dislodge items (Figure 2.11).

After removing the moistened lap pad from the oral cavity, the airway above the endotracheal tube is suctioned to remove any additional fluid. Before recovery from anesthesia, a complete oral exam and dental probing is recommended to rule out dental disease as a cause for nasal discharge (Figure 2.12).

Laryngoscopy

Laryngoscopy can be performed as an isolated procedure or as the preliminary assessment of the airway before a transoral tracheal wash or bronchoscopy. An appropriate anesthetic protocol must be devised that provides a light plane of anesthesia and preserves laryngeal function. While multiple agents are appropriate for use, the key feature is to have spontaneous and vigorous respirations. An assistant is required to identify inspiratory efforts so that the examiner can insure coordination of laryngeal abduction with inspiration. If the

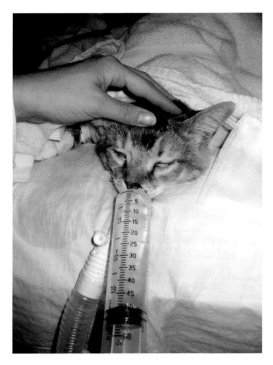

Figure 2.10. Nasal flush can be performed by inserting a syringe tip into the nostril and injecting pulses of chilled saline through each nostril. The animal must be intubated and have a moistened lap pad placed in the oral cavity to protect against aspiration.

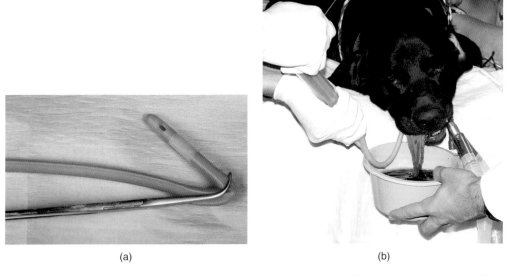

(a)   (b)

Figure 2.11. Right-angle forceps can be used to place a Foley catheter above the soft palate (a). After the balloon is inflated, copious nasal flush can be used to dislodge foreign material or exudate into a collection bowl (b).

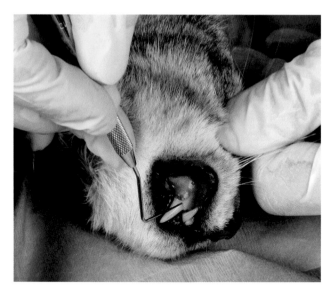

Figure 2.12.   A periodontal probe is inserted along the gum lines surrounding each tooth after imaging and rhinoscopy have been completed. Pockets >1 mm depth in the cat and >1–3 mm depth in the dog could result in clinically significant nasal disease due to tracking of bacteria up the tooth root into the nasal cavity.

plane of anesthesia is too deep, one to two boluses of doxapram (0.5–1.0 mg/kg) can be used to stimulate respirations (Miller et al. 2002).

Laryngoscopy includes the assessment of function as well as examination of all structures in the area of the rima glottis, including the soft palate, tonsils, laryngeal aditus, and saccules (Figure 2.13). The larynx is inspected for edema, hyperemia, or accumulation of secretions,

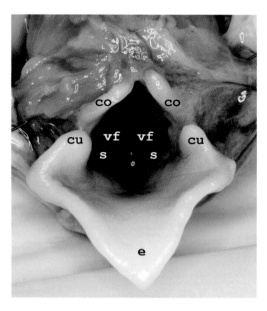

Figure 2.13.   Necropsy image of the larynx showing the corniculate processes of the arytenoids (co), vocal folds (vf), cuneiform processes of the arytenoids (cu), saccules (s), and epiglottis (e).

any of which could indicate injury due to excessive airflow, acid reflux, or lower airway inflammation. Eversion of laryngeal saccules is a common sign of obstruction to airflow in the upper airways (see Chapter 4). Because they are membranous tissue, saccules are very responsive to manipulation and may become more swollen as the upper airway evaluation continues. In the normal dog, the soft palate should not overlap with the epiglottis more than a few millimeters. Tonsils should be within their crypts; enlargement or eversion is suggestive of inflammation or irritation.

Bronchoscopy

Bronchoscopy is one of the most useful techniques for providing a diagnosis in animals with airway or lung disease. It can define the location, grade, and extent of tracheal ring flattening for planning stabilization through surgery or stent implantation, identify protrusion of the dorsal tracheal membrane into the tracheal lumen, document tracheal inflammation or irritation, visualize intrathoracic bronchial or airway collapse, and allow collection of bronchoalveolar lavage fluid to determine the contribution of small airway disease to respiratory signs.

Significant complications that can be encountered after bronchoscopy are worsened cough or increased airway obstruction. These occur most commonly in dogs that have severe tracheal collapse or bronchomalacia because irritation of the airway potentiates a cough, and suppression of respiratory effort by anesthetic agents allows passive collapse of diseased large and small airways. Excessive stress that induces cough and respiratory distress is particularly troublesome. Coughing can be partly alleviated by administering dilute lidocaine (approximately 1 mL of 1% lidocaine for a small dog) through the bronchoscope at the carina at the end of the procedure. Subcutaneous terbutaline (0.01 mg/kg) may improve respirations in dogs with collapsed airways, and recovery in an oxygen-enriched environment can lessen respiratory distress. Bronchospasm can be a particular problem in the cat with inflammatory airway disease that has severe cough and respiratory distress. Terbutaline should be given subcutaneously prior to the procedure at 0.01 mg/kg BID–TID to produce airway smooth muscle relaxation and reduce complications. Aerosolized albuterol can be given through the endotracheal tube at the end of the procedure if injectable terbutaline is not available.

General anesthesia is required for bronchoscopy to suppress coughing and laryngospasm, to allow examination of the airways without inducing trauma, and to protect the endoscope. Bronchoscopy can be performed using gas anesthesia if the animal is large enough for a 7- to 8-mm-size endotracheal tube. A special T adapter is used to pass the scope through the endotracheal tube while administering anesthetic gas and venting expired gases (Figure 2.14). In small dogs and cats, jet ventilation is typically used to provide oxygenation through bulk flow because placement of the scope through a small endotracheal tube would lead to obstruction and build up of CO_2.

Virtually all animals undergoing bronchoscopy suffer respiratory embarrassment. Prior to bronchoscopy, patients are preoxygenated with a facemask, and an anesthetic protocol is chosen that avoids excessive cardiopulmonary depression. Animals are placed in sternal recumbency and two mouth gags are in place throughout the procedure to protect the bronchoscope. The normal trachea appears round to oval with minimal laxity in the dorsal tracheal membrane (Figure 2.15). At the carina, bifurcation in the left and right mainstem bronchi provides a reliable landmark for assessing location within the airways

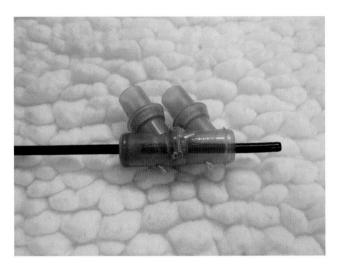

Figure 2.14.   Two endotracheal tube adapters have been fused together to create a T adapter that allows administration of anesthetic gas during bronchoscopy with a 5.0-mm fiberoptic endoscope. Oxygen and anesthetic gas are administered through the distal port and exhaust tubing is attached to the proximal port.

(Figure 2.16). Normal airways appear round to oval in shape, demonstrate little change in shape or diameter throughout respiration, have minimal secretions, and are pale pink in color (Figure 2.17). All accessible airways should be evaluated and abnormal regions with mucosal hyperemia or mucus accumulation should be identified as sites for bronchoalveolar lavage. If an obviously abnormal site is not visualized, the right middle lobe or caudal

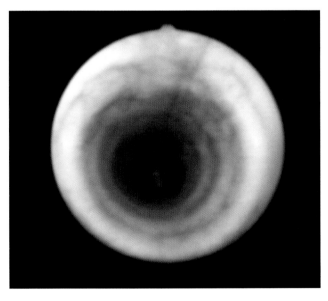

Figure 2.15.   Endoscopic view of the canine trachea. The notch at the top of the image is dorsal and the carina can be visualized in the distance.

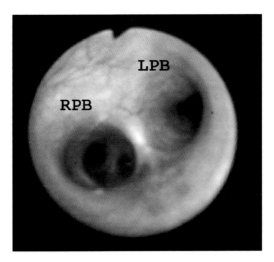

Figure 2.16. Endoscopic view of the carina illustrating the openings into the left principal bronchus (LPB) and right principal bronchus (RPB).

portion of the left cranial lobe are often worthwhile sites to lavage because they are ventrally oriented and tend to accumulate secretions.

After examining all visible airways, the scope is withdrawn from the airways, the outside is wiped with saline-soaked gauze pads, and the biopsy channel is flushed with sterile saline. On the second entry to the airway, the scope should be kept in the center of the airways to limit upper airway and mucosal contamination when approaching the site for lavage. Success in achieving a diagnostic bronchoalveolar lavage will depend on the ability to wedge the bronchoscope gently into a small airway and isolate a segment of alveolar

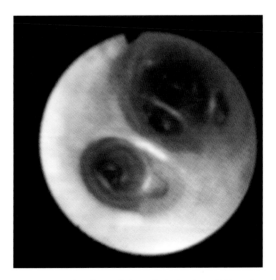

Figure 2.17. Distal airway openings in the dog exhibit relatively sharp bifurcations into round to oval airway openings. The epithelial surface is smooth.

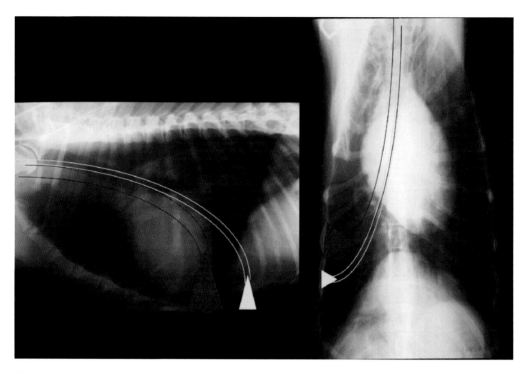

Figure 2.18. Bronchoalveolar lavage is performed by gently wedging the bronchoscope into the smallest airway possible. The volume of the region lavaged will depend on the size of the scope and the size of the animal.

volume (Figure 2.18). The goal is to flood this small wedge of lung with sterile lavage fluid, float the resident inflammatory cells, and gently aspirate back the fluid. The volume of fluid used depends on the size of the scope in relation to the size of the animal, experience of the operator, underlying disease process and degree of respiratory compromise (Table 2.4). If the fluid has been in contact with the alveolar space, it will be foamy because of the presence of surfactant. Flocculent material is usually mucus from bronchial contamination.

Table 2.4. General guidelines for performing bronchoalveolar lavage

Scope Size	Animal Size	milliliters per aliquot
2.8–3.8 mm outer diameter	Cats	3–5 mL
	Dogs <6 kg	5–10 mL
4.9–5.5 mm outer diameter	Dogs	15–20 mL

Note: For scopes >6 mm, consider passing sterile polypropylene tubing through the biopsy channel to wedge for BAL rather than using only the channel. Use of 15–20 mL/aliquot should be sufficient. Beware that the tubing can puncture the airway if extended with force.

Thoracocentesis

Thoracocentesis is performed as a diagnostic and therapeutic technique. It can be done before radiographs are performed when physical examination suggests a pleural disorder and the animal is in distress, or after radiographs when pleural space disease is confirmed. The region of the seventh to eighth intercostal space is clipped and scrubbed in the ventral one-third for fluid and in the dorsal one-third of the chest for air. A 20- or 22-gauge butterfly needle is adequate for use in small dogs and cats when small pleural effusion or mild pneumothorax is present. A fenestrated 14–18-gauge catheter with extension set works well for larger dogs and can allow relatively rapid removal of large pleural effusions. Prior to entering the chest, an extension set, three-way stopcock and syringe should be assembled and ready for use to limit introduction of air into the pleural space after penetration with the needle or catheter. A large bowl, EDTA and red top tubes, and a culturette swab should also be readily available to allow efficient specimen collection. In some animals, sedation is needed to perform a chest tap safely. Whenever possible, it is useful to have three people available to perform a chest tap.

A sterile preparation of the lateral thorax is completed and a site on the chest wall is chosen high on the wall for air and low for fluid. The needle or catheter is advanced through tented skin and then walked off the cranial border of the rib to penetrate the pleural space at a perpendicular angle. This will avoid the vessels and nerves lying along the caudal rib margin. As soon as the pleura has been penetrated, the needle or catheter is directed downward to avoid injury to the lung parenchyma (Figure 2.19). The needle stylet is held stationery while catheter is advanced into the thorax over the needle. When the catheter is fully in the chest, the needle is withdrawn, and the extension set is rapidly attached.

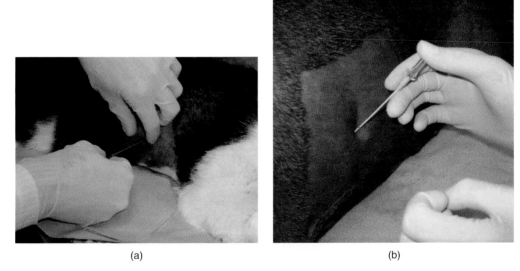

(a)   (b)

Figure 2.19.   To initiate thoracocentesis (a), the skin is tented and the catheter with needle is inserted perpendicularly between the rib spaces. After the pleural space has been entered (b), the needle is directed ventrally and the catheter is advanced fully into the chest while the needle is held stationery.

Fine-Needle Lung Aspiration and Biopsy

FNA of the lung is a suitable technique for evaluating diffuse interstitial or alveolar disorders or peripheral mass lesions within the thorax. It can be performed as a blind technique or with ultrasound guidance. However, because it can be associated with pneumothorax or hemothorax, careful patient selection is advised to limit complications. In animals that are not severely tachypneic or hyperpneic, percutaneous FNA of the lung can be performed safely and with minimal sedation. A small region of the chest is shaved and minor surgical preparation is completed. A 23–27-gauge three-fourths to 1 and half-inch needle attached to a 3-mL syringe filled with air is passed perpendicularly through the skin and subcutaneous tissue cranial to the border of the rib into the lung parenchyma. It is inserted back and forth gently and quickly; then the needle and syringe are removed together for preparation of cytologic specimens. The syringe is detached from the needle and filled with air, and contents of the needle hub are gently sprayed onto a slide or cover slip for cytologic examination and Gram staining. If aspiration with an empty syringe fails to yield material, the syringe can be filled with 0.5–1 mL of sterile saline, and the aspirated material is suspended in the saline for a cytospin preparation. Even when the sample appears to be of low cellularity, cytopathology is recommended to detect cellular atypia or inflammation.

Percutaneous lung biopsy can be obtained with use of an ultrasound guided biopsy needle in the anesthetized patient. This is performed more commonly in dogs than in cats. A surgical preparation is performed, and a 16–18-gauge Temno™ biopsy needle (Cardinal Health, Dublin, OH) is guided into the lesion to obtain a 2-cm core tissue sample for histopathology (Figure 2.20). After either aspiration or biopsy, the animal should be placed in lateral recumbency with the side of the aspiration facing downward for 15–30 minutes to promote the development of a clot or seal at the aspiration site. Radiographs or ultrasound should be performed to screen for hemorrhage or pneumothorax. An increase in respiratory rate or effort or detection of absent lung sounds would indicate the need for early intervention.

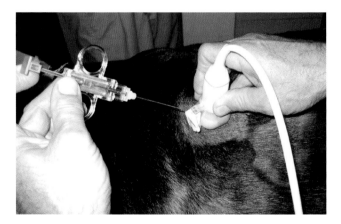

Figure 2.20. Ultrasound guidance is used to obtain a lung biopsy using a Temno biopsy needle. (Courtesy of Mr. Tom Baker, University of California, Davis.)

Sample Analysis

Nasal Cytology

Nasal cytology can be performed by pressing a microscope slide directly onto the nose of an animal or by obtaining material with a cotton swab and spreading it onto a slide. It is noninvasive and inexpensive; however, there are substantial limitations to the amount of information obtained from this test. Its primary usefulness is in the diagnosis of nasal fungal infection with cryptococcosis (see Chapter 4). Accuracy in the diagnosis of nasal aspergillosis or neoplasia is poor unless an endoscopically obtained sample from a fungal plaque or from a mass lesion is examined cytologically (De Lorenzi et al. 2006).

Nasal Culture

Bacterial culture of nasal discharge is not recommended. In fact, since most infections in the nose are secondary rather than primary, the value of culturing a deep nasal flush or nasal biopsy can also be questioned because of the difficulty in distinguishing normal flora from pathogens or opportunistic invaders. Interpretation of bacterial cultures is more difficult in animals that have been on multiple courses of antibiotic trials because this tends to favor development of resistant species. Despite this, bacterial culture from a deep nasal swab or flush can provide some direction for antibiotic therapy, particularly in cats with chronic rhinosinusitis. A deep nasal flush is obtained by inserting an 8-French red rubber catheter halfway into the rostral nasal cavity, occluding the soft palate digitally, and instilling and aspirating 2 mL of sterile saline. Culture for aerobic bacteria and *Mycoplasma* spp. is recommended.

A recent study on the utility of fungal cultures in the diagnosis of canine nasal aspergillosis reported moderate sensitivity (77%) but high specificity (100%) (Pomrantz et al. 2007). In that study, the material submitted for culture was from a visualized fungal plaque and therefore, a low number of false-positive values would be expected. In cases of cryptococcoisis, culture and speciation can be helpful in determining the epidemiology of the infection, although subclinical colonization of the nasal cavity has been reported in 7–14% of dogs and cats (Malik et al. 1997).

Nasal Histology

Histopathology provides the diagnosis of aspergillosis in cases in which a plaque lesion has been sampled by direct visualization; however, a random sampling of the nasal mucosa may not contain fungal elements, leading to a false-negative biopsy sample. Neoplasia can be difficult to confirm because a rim of necrosis and inflammation often surrounds neoplastic cells. In some instances, neoplastic cells can be documented in histopathology from a mass in the nasopharynx but are not found within the nasal cavity. This seems particularly common in feline nasal/nasopharyngeal lymphoma.

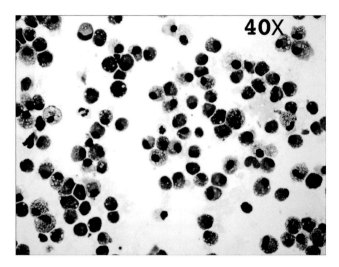

Figure 2.21.   Cytocentrifuge of a normal bronchoalveolar lavage sample (40×) reveals primarily macrophages and occasional neutrophils and eosinophils.

Airway Wash Cytology

Normal tracheal wash cytology is composed of ciliated columnar to cuboidal epithelial cells and rare macrophages or inflammatory cells. Normal bronchoalveolar lavage cytology contains primarily of alveolar macrophages (65–75%), with 5–10% neutrophils, lymphocytes, and eosinophils (although in a cat, 18–25% eosinophils can be normal) (Figure 2.21). Normal macrophages can exhibit variable appearances depending upon the stimuli present within the lung. Active macrophages contain intracellular inclusions, may appear foamy, and may be engulfing granulocytes or particulate matter in comparison to quiescent macrophages. Normal cell counts have been reported for the dog and cat and are approximately 300–400 cells/μL. Higher cell counts and/or altered percentage of cells present within the lavage fluid are indicative of lower respiratory tract disease.

The presence of macrophages in conjunction with increased numbers of neutrophils, plus or minus lymphocytes and eosinophils, characterizes pyogranulomatous inflammation. This generally occurs in response to significant airway insult and is usually due to chronic disease such as chronic aspiration pneumonia, smoke inhalation, bronchiectasis, or neoplasia. Fungal disease can also result in pyogranulomatous inflammation and samples should be closely screened for cytologic evidence of fungal organisms (see Chapter 6). Suppurative inflammation is characterized by >10% neutrophils and can represent pure inflammation as in chronic bronchitis and feline bronchial disease or may be an indicator of infection as with pneumonia. The finding of degenerate neutrophils containing intracellular bacteria is a reliable indicator of bacterial pneumonia.

Eosinophilic inflammation is a characteristic of feline bronchial asthma and can also be found with airway parasitism due to *Aelurostrongylus*, *Capillaria*, or *Paragonimus*, in heartworm disease, or with larval migration of gastrointestinal parasites (*Toxocara*). Airway eosinophilia is a prominent feature of eosinophilic bronchopneumopathy in dogs.

Hemorrhagic inflammation can be found with rodenticide intoxication (vitamin K antagonists), heartworm or *Paragonimus* infection, foreign body, trauma, or erosive neoplasms.

Evidence of previous airway hemorrhage (indicated by macrophages ingesting red blood cells or hemosiderin-laden macrophages) can be found in some dogs with congestive heart failure, lung neoplasia, or with exercise-induced pulmonary hemorrhage.

In rare instances, malignant cells may exfoliate into the airways with pulmonary carcinoma (primary or metastatic) or in pulmonary involvement with lymphoma and be detected in bronchoalveolar lavage fluid. Characteristics of malignancy are similar to those in other tissues, including loss of contact inhibition, variation in cell size or nuclear size and shape, increased nuclear-to-cytoplasmic ratio, basophilia, multinucleate cells or frequent cells undergoing mitosis. Neoplastic transformation may be difficult to confirm because dysplastic changes associated with severe inflammation can mimic neoplastic change. In addition, some lung tumors have a necrotic center or may have infection in addition to neoplastic transformation, which can complicate interpretation of abnormal appearing cells or the presence of bacteria. Review of several samples may be required to confirm the presence of an underlying neoplasm. If a mass lesion is noted in the airway lumen during bronchoscopic examination, an endoscopic biopsy sample should be obtained.

Airway Culture

Positive bacterial and mycoplasmal cultures must be interpreted in conjunction with cytology. The presence of squamous cells or *Simonsiella* bacteria is suggestive of upper airway contamination. In these cases, it is not uncommon to observe growth of two to four types of aerobic bacteria (usually oral flora) with or without *Mycoplasma*. Intracellular bacteria and the presence of septic, suppurative inflammation are present with true bacterial infection. These are characterized by lack of squamous cells on cytology and a variably increased percentage of neutrophils, some of which contain bacteria. Since approximately one-third of healthy dogs and almost three-fourths of healthy cats can have positive tracheal cultures (Table 2.5), strict attention should be paid to upper airway contamination of BAL samples and appropriate interpretation of BAL cultures. Quantitative bacterial cultures provide evidence for bacterial infection when $>1.7 \times 10^3$ bacterial colony forming units per milliliter of fluid grow on culture. In addition, detection of more than two intracellular bacteria in any of 50 examined high-power fields is a reliable indicator of lower respiratory tract infection (Peeters et al. 2000). Lower respiratory tract infections are often characterized by culture of several species of bacteria with mixed bacteria reported in 43% cases in one study (Angus et al. 1997).

Pleural Fluid Analysis

Initial analysis on pleural fluid should always include a PCV, cell count, protein or specific gravity, and cytology. Smears may also be prepared for Gram staining. Additional diagnostic tests for systemic disease such as a complete blood count, chemistry panel, urinalysis, or echocardiogram can be chosen after the character of the pleural fluid is determined (Table 2.6). Additional tests to perform on pleural fluid include bacterial culture and susceptibility testing (aerobic and anaerobic cultures), protein electrophoresis, or a cholesterol/triglyceride ratio for the diagnosis of chylothorax.

Table 2.5. Lower respiratory tract flora found in healthy dogs and cats

Dogs (McKiernan 1984)	Cats (Dye 1996)
Bordetella	Acinetobacter
Corynebacterium	Bordetella
Escherichia coli	Corynebacterium
Enterobacter	Enterobacter
Klebsiella	Flavobacterium
Pasteurella	Klebsiella
Pseudomonas	Pasteurella
Staphylococcus	Staphylococcus
Streptococcus	α-Streptococcus
Mycoplasma	

Pleural Fluid Culture

When an exudative pleural effusion is obtained (protein >3 g/dL and cells >5000/µL), samples of pleural fluid should be cultured for both aerobes and anaerobes. In a retrospective study of pyothorax (Walker et al. 2000), bacteria were isolated from 45 of 47 cats (96%) and were visible on cytology in 41 of 45 samples (91%). Obligate anaerobes were present

Table 2.6. Characteristics of pleural fluid

	Protein (g/dL)	Cell Count (per µL)	Etiology
Transudate	≪ 1.5	≪ 1,000	Hypoalbuminemia
Modified transudate	<2.5	500–2,500	Right heart failure Pericardial disease Neoplasia Hernia
Exudate	>3.0	>5,000	FIP Neoplasia Hernia Lung lobe torsion Pyothorax
Chylous	>2.5	>500	Idiopathic Cardiomyopathy Heartworm disease Neoplasia Lung lobe torsion
Hemorrhagic	>3.0	>1,000	Trauma Coagulopathy Neoplasia Lung lobe torsion

in 40 of 45 samples (89%), and a mixture of obligate anaerobes and facultative organisms was found in 20 of 45 (44%) of culture positive cats. An average of 2.1 species of obligate anaerobic bacteria and 1.2 species of aerobic bacteria were isolated in cats. In dogs, bacteria were isolated from 47 of 51 samples (92%) and were visible on cytology in 32 of 47 samples (68%). Bacteria included obligate anaerobes in 17 of 47 positive samples (36%), and mixed obligate anaerobes and facultative organisms in 17 of 47 samples (36%). An average of 2.4 species of obligate anaerobic bacteria and 1.6 species of aerobic bacteria were isolated in dogs. In dogs, enteric organisms were the most common aerobic bacteria isolated, while in cats, *Pasteurella* species were isolated most commonly. Similar anaerobes were isolated from cats and dogs, with *Peptostreptococcus*, *Bacteroides*, and *Fusobacterium* isolated most commonly.

References

Angus JC, Jang SS, Hirsh DC. Microbiological study of transtracheal aspirates from dogs with suspected lower respiratory tract disease: 264 cases (1989–1995). J Am Vet Med Assoc. 1997; 210: 55–58.

De Lorenzi D, Bonfanti U, Masserdotti C, et al. Diagnosis of canine nasal aspergillosis by cytological examination: a comparison of four different collection techniques. J Small Anim Pract. 2006; 47: 316–319.

Dye JA, McKiernan BC, Rozanski EA, et al. Bronchopulmonary disease in the cat: historical, physical, radiographic, clinicopathologic, and pulmonary functional evaluation of 24 affected and 15 healthy cats. J Vet Intern Med. 1996; 10: 385–400.

Foster SF, Martin P, Braddock JA, Malik R. A retrospective analysis of feline bronchoalveolar lavage cytology and microbiology. J Fel Med Surg. 2004; 6: 189–198.

Hawkins EC, Berry CR. Use of a modified stomach tube for bronchoalveolar lavage in dogs. J Am Vet Med Assoc. 1999; 215: 1635–1629.

Hawkins EC, Stoskopf SK, Levy J, et al. Cytologic characterization of bronchoalveolar lavage fluid collected through an endotracheal tube in cats. Am J Vet Res. 1994; 55: 795–802.

Malik R, Wigney DI, Muir DB, Love DN. Asymptomatic carriage of *Crtyptoccus neoformans* in the nasal cavity of dogs and cats. J Med Vet Mycol. 1997; 35: 27–31.

McKiernan BC, Smith AR, Kissil M. Bacterial isolates from the lower trachea of clinically healthy dogs. J Am Anim Hosp Assoc. 1982; 20: 139–142.

Miller CJ, McKiernan BC, Pace J, Fettman MJ. The effects of doxapram hydrochloride (dopram-V) on laryngeal function in healthy dogs. J Vet Intern Med. 2002; 16: 524–528.

Peeters DE, McKiernan BC, Weisiger RM, et al. Quantitative bacterial cultures and cytological examination of bronchoalveolar lavage specimens in dogs. J Vet Intern Med. 2000; 14: 534–541.

Pomrantz JS, Johnson LR, Nelson RW, Wisner ER. Comparison of serologic evaluation via agar gel immunodiffusion and fungal culture of tissue for diagnosis of nasal aspergillosis in dogs. J Am Vet Med Assoc. 2007; 230: 1319–1323.

Walker AL, Jang SS, Hirsh DW. Bacteria associated with pyothorax of dogs and cats: 98 cases (1989–1998). J Am Vet Med Assoc. 2000; 216: 359–363.

Respiratory Therapeutics 3

Drug Therapy

Antibiotics for Upper Respiratory Tract Disease

Empiric antibiotic therapy is often used in animals with presumed respiratory infection prior to obtaining definitive information on the bacteria involved because susceptibility results take 2–5 days to become available or because of an inability to obtain an appropriate sample. Treatment of presumed infections of the upper or lower respiratory tract requires knowledge of the normal flora found in these locations as well as an understanding of the species most likely to be pathogenic. In kittens with acute (likely viral) upper respiratory disease, flora of the upper respiratory tract (*Staphylococcus, Streptococcus, Pasteurella, Bordetella*, and anaerobes) may overwhelm local defenses and colonize the nasal cavity, leading to clinical signs of sneezing and mucopurulent nasal discharge. Antibiotics are commonly administered for 1–2 weeks to kittens with acute upper respiratory infection to reduce bacterial numbers and decrease bacterial invasion of epithelium damaged by viral infection. Fortunately, many commonly encountered bacterial strains remain susceptible to amoxicillin–clavulanic acid or to fluoroquinolones (Dossin et al. 1998). Azithromycin also has clinical efficacy for acute feline upper respiratory tract infection. It is important to remember that penicillin derivatives are ineffective against *Mycoplasma* spp., a cell-wall-deficient bacteria. Because this organism can be found in acute feline upper respiratory disease, use of doxycycline or a fluoroquinolone would be appropriate.

In chronic upper respiratory tract disease in the cat, aerobic bacterial infection is a common complication (Johnson et al. 2005). The chronic disease is typically characterized by devitalization of tissue with accumulation of inflammatory products, and resolution of disease is difficult to achieve. Doxycycline and azithromycin are attractive drugs to use in such cases because they possess anti-inflammatory effects as well as antimicrobial action. A fluoroquinolone is a rational antibiotic choice for some cases because these drugs have excellent efficacy against most Gram-negative bacteria and *Mycoplasma*. However, a high dose may be required for successful treatment of *Pseudomonas* infections, and this is not advisable in cats because of potential retinal toxicity. Newer fluoroquinolones (pradofloxacin and premafloxacin) also have some efficacy against anaerobic organisms. For cats with underlying osteomyelitis or suspected anaerobic infections, a drug such as clindamycin could be more effective in controlling clinical signs since it penetrates bone tissue.

When treating the bacterial component of feline upper respiratory tract disease, consideration should be given to using a long course (4–6 weeks) of antibiotics to achieve maximal control of bacterial numbers. In some cases, chronic use of antibiotics is required.

Bacterial involvement in canine inflammatory rhinitis appears to be less prominent than in the feline syndrome, although few studies have evaluated isolation rates in dogs with nasal discharge (Windsor et al. 2004). Secondary bacterial infection can develop in dogs that have been treated for nasal aspergillosis infections because of destruction of turbinates and loss of normal nasal defense mechanisms. In those cases, 7–10 days of any broad-spectrum antibiotic (e.g., amoxicillin-clavulanic acid) can help alleviate nasal discharge, although it will often recur.

Antibiotics for Lower Respiratory Tract Disease

Lower respiratory tract infection can be life-threatening and antibiotics should be based on culture and susceptibility testing whenever possible. However, when culture results are pending or when airway sampling is not clinically feasible, initial antibiotic choices must consider the likely species involved and reported susceptibility patterns of commonly encountered bacteria (Table 3.1).

Appropriate therapy for bacterial respiratory infection often requires antibiotics directed at Gram-negative and -positive aerobes, anaerobes, and *Mycoplasma* organisms. Rational choices for initial therapy of newly diagnosed infections (before final culture results are available) would include enrofloxacin with a penicillin drug, metronidazole, or clindamycin. Ticarcillin, a carboxypenicillin formulated only for intravenous use, is a valuable drug to employ in early treatment of pneumonia. It has improved efficacy in treatment of *Pseudomonas* infection as well as anaerobic infections; however, it is ineffective against *Mycoplasma* spp. Ticarcillin-clavulanate bypasses beta-lactamase resistance mediated by plasmids. Anaerobic susceptibility testing is rarely performed because organisms are difficult to grow on susceptibility plates however most are sensitive to penicillins. *Bacteroides* spp. are relatively resistant to clindamycin therapy (Jang et al. 1997) and penicillin, metronidazole or chloramphenicol would be better choices when infection with this anaerobe is documented. Chloramphenicol has excellent efficacy against a number of organisms commonly implicated in respiratory infection; however, use of this drug may be associated with central nervous system depression, anorexia, vomiting, or bone marrow suppression. Lower respiratory tract infections require 2–6 weeks of antibiotic treatment, and long-term therapy should be determined by results of bacterial culture and sensitivity in complicated cases.

Azalides (azithromycin and clarithromycin) have efficacy against Gram-positive and Gram-negative organisms and *Mycoplasma*. These drugs have the advantage of producing high and prolonged tissue levels, typically resulting in enhanced bacterial killing. Recent

Table 3.1. Gram-stain characteristics and antibiotic susceptibility for common bacteria

Organism	Gram Stain	First-Line Antibiotics
Bordetella	Negative coccobacillus	Aerosolized gentocin Doxycycline Chloramphenicol
Escherichia coli	Negative rod	Fluoroquinolones Ceftizoxime, Ceftiofur Amikacin, Gentocin Trimethoprim-sulfa
Klebsiella	Negative rod	Fluoroquinolones Amikacin, Gentocin Ceftizoxime, Ceftiofur, Clavamox Trimethoprim-Sulfa
Pseudomonas	Negative rod	Fluoroquinolones Carbenicillin Amikacin Cephalosporin and gentocin
Pasteurella	Negative rod	Clavamox Chloramphenicol Cephalosporin Trimethoprim-sulfa
Streptococcus	Positive coccus	Amoxicillin–clavulanic acid Ampicillin Cephalosporin
Staphylococcus	Positive coccus	Methacillin Cloxacin Cephalosporin
Mycoplasma		Doxycycline Chloramphenicol Fluoroquinolones Azithromycin
Anaerobes	Positive or negative	Clindamycin Metronidazole Penicillins Chloramphenicol Cephalosporin

studies in the cat showed variability in drug half-life, but relatively high bioavailability (58%) and sustained accumulation of drug in tissues after a single oral dose of 5.4 mg/kg (Hunter et al. 1995). The efficacy of azithromycin in feline respiratory diseases is not yet known; however, its pharmacokinetic properties and pulmonary penetration could prove valuable in the treatment of respiratory infections. In general, antibiotic treatment should be used for immediate control of infectious lung disease; however, in some situations, chronic antibiotic therapy or intermittent pulse therapy with antibiotics may be required to control clinical signs in dogs with bronchiectasis and animals with ciliary dyskinesia. In these disorders, mucus accumulation with trapping of bacteria in secretions can result in severe and

Table 3.2.   Side effects of commonly used antibiotics

Penicillins and cephalosporins	Hypersensitivity response
	Immune mediated hemolytic anemia
Trimethoprim-sulfa	Keratoconjuctivitis sicca
	Folate deficient anemia
	Decreased thyroid function
	Arthropathy (black and tan dogs)
Enrofloxacin	Retinal toxicity (cats)
	Cartilage injury (immature animals)
Metronidazole	Neurotoxicity
Doxycycline	Esophageal stricture
	Photosensitivity
	Hepatotoxicity
Chloramphenicol	Bone marrow toxicity
Aminoglycosides	Renal toxicity
	Ototoxicity

recurrent pneumonia. The antibiotic chosen should have proper efficacy, should penetrate the airway, and should be relatively free of side effects.

If a fluoroquinolone is needed in an animal that is being treated with theophylline, it is important to note that this class of drug inhibits the metabolism of theophylline, and use of the two drugs together results in toxic plasma levels (Intorre et al. 1995). At least 30% reduction in theophylline dose is recommended when a fluoroquinolone is used concurrently.

Side Effects of Antibiotics

Virtually any antibiotic can be associated with gastrointestinal complaints of vomiting, diarrhea, or anorexia. Other important side effects are listed in Table 3.2.

Antifungal Therapy

Fungal infection in the respiratory tract most commonly involves *Cryptococcus neoformans* or *Aspergillus fumigatus* in the nasal cavity of cats or dogs, respectively, and *Histoplasma capsulatum*, *Blastomyces dermatitidis*, or *Coccidioides immitis* organisms in the lower respiratory tract. Nasal aspergillosis is a special condition, which appears to respond best to extensive debridement of fungal plaques and topical antifungal therapy (see Chapter 4). When treating fungal respiratory tract infection, long-term therapy (6 weeks to over 12 months) must be anticipated. Depending on the severity of disease, the presence of concurrent illness and the initial response to therapy, fungistatic or fungicidal agents administered orally or parenterally should be chosen (Table 3.3).

The azoles (itraconazole, fluconazole, voriconazole, posaconazole) are fungistatic agents that inhibit P450 enzymes involved in synthesis of ergosterol, a key component of the fungal cell wall. Itraconazole (Sporanox®, Janssen Pharmaceuticals, Inc.) can be used as

Table 3.3. Antifungal drug therapy

Drug	Formulation	Dose	Mechanism	Indications	Side Effects
Fluconazole	50-, 100-, 200-mg tablets	2.5–5 mg/kg daily to BID	Static	Best for CNS penetration. May be the best drug for histoplasmosis in cats	Generic available Renally excreted
Itraconazole	100 capsules 5 mg/mL oral solution	5 mg/kg daily to BID 1.0–1.5 mg/kg of the liquid	Static	May be used alone or in combination with Amphotericin B	Liver toxicity Dermatotoxicity
Voriconazole	50- and 200-mg tablets 40 mg/mL oral suspension 10 mg/mL solution for i.v. use	2.5–10 mg/kg PO daily to BID Dilute to 5 mg/mL or less and infuse at a maximum rate of 3 mg/kg/hour over 1–2 hours	Static	Any susceptible fungal infection. Consider for nasal aspergillosis that has breached the cribriform plate	Liver toxicity
Posaconazole	40 mg/mL oral suspension		Static	Any susceptible fungal infection. Consider for nasal aspergillosis that has breached the cribriform plate	
Terbinafine	250-mg tablet	One-fourth of 250-mg tablet daily (cat)	Static		
Flucytosine	250-mg capsule 75 mg/mL oral suspension	30–50 mg/kg PO TID–QID	Static	For CNS infection with *Cryptococcus* in combination with an azole.	
Amphotericin B	50-mg vial	0.5–1.0 mg/kg i.v. EOD to total dose of 5–14 mg/kg	Cidal	Fungicidal treatment of fungal pneumonia	Nephrotoxic Drug fever Thrombophlebitis
Amphotericin B Lipid complex	5-mg/mL in a 20 mL vial	0.5–1.0 mg/kg i.v. EOD to a total dose of 10–20 mg/kg	Cidal	Fungicidal treatment of fungal pneumonia	Less/no nephrotoxicity Drug fever

sole therapy for nasal or pulmonary fungal infection or can be used following amphotericin B for sustained control of disease. Itraconazole is excreted by the liver, and side effects of therapy include hepatic toxicity, dermatotoxicity, and anorexia. Fluconazole is available in generic form. It is renally excreted thus a reduced dosage is recommended for animals with renal insufficiency. Voriconazole (Vfend®, Pfizer) and posaconazole (Noxafil®, Schering-Plough) are new triazoles with improved antifungal activity.

Terbinafine is an allylamine fungistatic agent that is thought to act through inhibition of squalene epoxidase during the synthesis of ergosterol for the fungal cell membrane. Side effects are apparently rare. Flucytosine is a pyrimidine analog that also inhibits fungal synthesis. It is used only in combination with other antifungal agents because it is a relatively weak antifungal and because of rapid development of resistance. It is indicated primarily for treatment of central nervous system cryptococcosis.

Amphotericin B is a fungicidal drug that creates breaks in the fungal cell membrane. Because it is highly nephrotoxic, aggressive diuresis with 0.9% saline (20–40 mg/kg over 1–3 hours) is recommended prior to administration. After saline diuresis, the infusion line is flushed with 5% dextrose to avoid precipitation of the amphotericin in saline. A central vein is recommended to avoid thrombophlebitis, and the drug should be protected from light during administration. A test dose of 0.5 mg/kg in 5% dextrose solution is administered intravenously over 5–6 hours on the first day of therapy. Body temperature is continually measured during the infusion because of the likelihood of a drug fever. On the day after administration, renal parameters are measured, and if values are within normal limits, a dose of 1.0 mg/kg can be administered on the following day. This regimen is continued until renal insufficiency necessitates discontinuation of therapy or until fungal disease is under control, which may require cumulative dosages of 5–14 mg/kg. If residual disease is suspected or the animal can no longer tolerate intravenous therapy, oral azole treatment is used for continual control of disease. Amphotericin B can also be administered subcutaneously in fractious animals, those that cannot be hospitalized, or those that cannot be treated with oral medications. Amphotericin B at a dose of 0.5–0.8 mg/kg is diluted in 400–500 mL of 0.45% NaCl/2.5% dextrose and administered subcutaneously two to three times weekly until disease has resolved.

To reduce the likelihood of renal insufficiency, administration of amphotericin B lipid complex is recommended. The drug is given as a 20–30-minute infusion of 0.5–1.0 mg/kg and pretreatment with saline diuresis is not a requirement. This drug is more expensive than standard amphotericin B and is formulated in a single-use vial.

Antiviral Therapy

Viruses (feline herpes virus-1: FHV-1; feline calicivirus: FCV) have been implicated as major etiologic agents in acute feline upper respiratory disease. Because clinical signs are generally self-limiting, specific diagnostic tests to identify infecting organisms are rarely performed and antiviral therapy is rarely used. In the chronic disease syndrome, presence of the upper respiratory viruses is poorly correlated with disease status. Clinical signs may be due to direct cytopathic effects mediated by the virus or due to the host's immunologic response to infection. Lower respiratory tract disease due to viral infection is less common but may occur with some upper respiratory tract viruses or due to infection with the mutated coronavirus (feline infectious peritonitis virus: FIP). Many respiratory manifestations of feline infectious peritonitis virus are related to the host's immunologic response and subsequent vasculitis, and definitive diagnosis of FIP remains difficult. Controversy surrounding viral pathogenesis of disease and diagnostic methods makes it difficult to determine whether antiviral therapy is warranted in suspect cases.

Efficacy of antiviral agents in clinical feline respiratory diseases has not been established, however, pharmacokinetics have been studied for some drugs. Acyclovir and valacyclovir, a prodrug of acyclovir, are not recommended because of poor efficacy against FHV-1 and unacceptable toxicity. The most promising drug for use against FHV-1-related ocular disease is famcyclovir, although this drug has not been evaluated specifically for chronic nasal disease in the cat. Supplementation with oral lysine (250–500 mg PO BID) might be helpful in kittens or cats with upper respiratory disease that is presumed to be viral in origin. Lysine competes with arginine in FHV-1 protein synthesis, and inhibition of synthetic activity decreases replication of the virus. Supplementation does not result in systemic arginine depletion and no side effects have been reported.

Viruses associated with canine infectious respiratory disease complex can cause severe pneumonia in dogs, however specific antiviral therapy has been investigated for use in canine viral pneumonias.

Glucocorticoids

Corticosteroids are indicated for long-term control of feline bronchial disease, chronic bronchitis, and canine eosinophilic lung disease. Corticosteroids reduce inflammation by inhibition of phospholipase A2, the enzyme responsible for the initial metabolism of arachidonic acid into inflammatory mediators. Corticosteroids also decrease migration of inflammatory cells into the airway, thus decreasing the concentration of granulocyte products and reactants (major basic protein, eosinophil cationic protein, reactive oxygen species), which perpetuate epithelial injury.

Short-acting oral steroids are preferred for treatment of inflammatory airway disease in the dog or the cat to allow an accurate titration of the dose that controls clinical signs while inducing minimal side effects. Prednisolone is the preferred steroid to use in the cat, while either prednisone or prednisolone can be used in the dog. Long-acting glucocorticoids such as dexamethasone, triamcinolone, and methylprednisolone acetate do not have a therapeutic advantage over prednisone, and use of a repositol steroid could result in waxing and waning of inflammation between injections that perpetuates disease. The duration and dose of corticosteroid therapy will depend upon the severity and chronicity of respiratory signs, the extent of the infiltrates on radiographs, and the degree of inflammation on cytology. An individualized approach to anti-inflammatory treatment is required for each case, with a gradual reduction in dose to the minimal level that controls clinical signs.

The length of therapy required to alleviate signs is unknown; however, long-term therapy (2–3 months for dogs with chronic bronchitis and 4–5 months for dogs with eosinophilic disease) can be anticipated in most cases. Discontinuation of medication may be possible, although many cats with inflammatory airway disease will require life-long medication continually or intermittently. If disease worsens during lowering of the dose, a return to the higher dose of glucocorticoid that controlled clinical signs is generally required. Alternately, treatment with inhaled steroids, bronchodilators, or antitussive agents can be added depending on the disease process (see later).

Bronchodilators

The two main classes of bronchodilators used in veterinary medicine are methylxanthine derivatives (theophylline) and beta-agonists. While these agents provide only mild relaxation of airway smooth muscle and bronchodilation, they can be clinically helpful in reducing signs in dogs or cats with bronchitis or in allowing a reduction in the dosage of glucocorticoid required to control signs.

Methylxanthines

Methylxanthine agents such as theophylline and aminophylline are used clinically as bronchodilators. Although known pharmacologically as a phosphodiesterase inhibitor, the dose of theophylline used clinically does not result in sufficient accumulation of cyclic adenosine monophosphate to cause smooth muscle relaxation. Current research suggests that the clinical effects of methylxanthines likely result from adenosine antagonism or from alterations in cellular sensitivity to calcium. Theophylline may provide other beneficial effects by increasing diaphragmatic muscle strength, improving pulmonary perfusion, reducing respiratory effort, and stimulating mucociliary clearance (in dogs, but not in cats). Studies evaluating pharmocokinetics of one brand of extended-release theophylline suggested a dose of 10 mg/kg PO every 12 hours in a dog and 15 or 19 mg/kg once daily in the evening for the cat to approximate the human therapeutic range of 10–20 mg/mL. (Bach et al. 2004, Guenther-Yenke et al. 2007). Most extended release theophylline products can be split in half once and will retain the extended release properties. It is unknown whether generic forms of sustained-release theophylline are bioequivalent to the form that has been studied; however, these products would be preferred over aminophylline, which is poorly bioavailable in dogs and cats.

Adverse effects of methylxanthines are likely related to adenosine antagonism and include gastrointestinal upset, tachycardia, and hyperexcitability. It is essential to individualize drug therapy because there is a wide variation in the dose that causes side effects. Theophylline metabolism is influenced by many factors, including fiber in the diet, smoke in the environment, congestive heart failure, and the use of other drugs. Because of concerns about metabolism and unknown bioavailability, a reduced dosage can be considered initially (5 mg/kg every 12 hours in a dog and 5–10 mg/kg once daily in the cat), and if the animal tolerates the drug, the dosage may be increased as needed.

Methylxanthines are relatively weak bronchodilators and while they may be beneficial for adjunctive therapy in control of clinical signs, they are not recommended for use in an acute or emergency situation.

Beta-agonists

Administration of a beta-2 agonist (terbutaline or albuterol) results in bronchodilation due to direct relaxation of airway smooth muscle, and intravenous terbutaline has been shown to reduce airway resistance acutely in cats with constricted airways (Dye et al. 1996). Preliminary pharmacokinetic studies have established the safety of the drug, and the recommended dose is 0.01 mg/kg parenterally or 0.625 mg/cat PO BID. Small dogs can receive 0.625–1.25 mg PO every 12 hours, medium-sized dogs are given 1.25–2.5 mg PO every 12 hours, and larger dogs receive 2.5–5 mg PO every 12 hours. Active bronchoconstriction does not play a role in canine chronic bronchitis as it does in a subset of cats with bronchitis; however, albuterol at 50 μg/kg PO every 8 hours was efficacious in reducing cough in almost half the dogs evaluated in a review of canine chronic bronchitis (Padrid et al. 1990). Interestingly, the bronchodilator also resulted in a reduction in the severity of the pulmonary infiltrate. Theoretically, chronic use of a beta-agonist can result in downregulation of beta-receptor density and decreased efficacy of the drug, although it is unclear if this is recognized clinically. As with methylxanthines, beta-agonists may result in excitability or tremors during initial therapy, but animals usually become accustomed to the drug. Beta-2 agonists can be administered orally and are widely available for inhaled therapy; however, prolonged use of specific forms of albuterol could potentially worsen airway inflammation (Reinero et al. 2009).

Mucolytics

Marked controversy exists concerning the utility of mucolytic agents in human medicine, and there is little information on the use or efficacy of these preparations in veterinary patients. Clinical experience suggests that some dogs and cats with excessive production of airway secretions associated with chronic infectious or inflammatory diseases may benefit from their use. Conditions that might respond to mucolytic agents include feline chronic rhinosinusitis, canine lymphoplasmacytic rhinitis, chronic bronchitis, bronchiectasis, and pneumonia-associated with production of viscous secretions (e.g., *Mycoplasma*).

Mucolytic/expectorant agents such as N-acetylcysteine, bromhexine, S-carboxy-methylcysteine, ambroxol, guaifenesin, and iodinated glycerol can thin the viscosity of mucin-containing secretions. These drugs act by a variety of mechanisms including breakage of disulfide bonds in airway mucoproteins, stimulation of serous airway secretions, or breakdown of acid mucopolysaccharide fibers in sputum. N-acetylcysteine and S-carboxymethylcysteine can be administered orally or by inhalation, although nebulization with N-acetylcysteine may result in bronchoconstriction or epithelial injury and this route is not routinely recommended. The rest of these agents are designed for oral use. N-acetylcysteine is reported to provide a variety of antioxidant and endothelial effects that might prove beneficial in respiratory patients. N-acetylcysteine is typically available in 600 mg capsules, and an empiric dose of 30–60 mg/kg (not to exceed 600 mg) PO BID–TID can be clinically efficacious in improving evacuation of mucus.

Antitussive Agents

The cough reflex is of major importance in animals because it serves the essential function of clearing secretions from the airway. Suppression of this reflex before resolution of inflammation can be deleterious because mucus can become trapped in small airways, and prolonged contact between inflammatory mediators in the mucus and epithelial cells perpetuates airway injury. If infection is present, cough suppression can lead to serious pneumonia. When clinical signs suggest that inflammation is resolving yet the cough persists, cough suppression is desirable because chronic coughing can lead to repeated airway injury and syncopal events. Cough suppressants are used almost exclusively in dogs rather than cats, and are often required in dogs with airway collapse or irritant tracheitis.

Over-the-counter dextromethorphan-containing compounds are only occasionally efficacious in some animals with airway disease. When more potent suppression of a dry cough is required, narcotic agents should be prescribed. Hydrocodone bitartrate (0.22 mg/kg PO every 6–12 hours) or butorphanol tartrate (0.5 mg/kg PO every 6–12 hours) can be used in dogs. These agents must be given at an interval that suppresses coughing without inducing excessive sedation. The drugs are initially given at a high dose several times daily and tapered to the lowest dose that controls clinical signs. Long-term therapy may be required in some patients; however, overuse should be avoided since tolerance can develop.

Routes of Administration

Parenteral Versus Enteral

For treatment of life-threatening disease, parenteral administration of a microbiocidal agent rather than a static drug provides optimal therapy. An exception to this might be the animal with severe pulmonary infiltrates associated with fungal pneumonia. Rapid killing of large numbers of organisms can lead to acute respiratory distress syndrome when an exuberant inflammatory response damages the alveolocapillary membrane, resulting in noncardiogenic pulmonary edema (see Chapter 8). In a severely affected animal with marked tachypnea and elevated work of breathing, consideration should be given to achieving a controlled kill of organisms with a static drug.

Parenteral administration of drugs is indicated for any animal with swallowing disorders, vomiting, or malabsorptive intestinal disease. Renal and hepatic function should be evaluated and monitored throughout therapy since many drugs (particularly antifungal medications) rely on renal or hepatic excretion for removal from the body or can cause organ dysfunction.

Nebulization

Nebulization can be used to hydrate airway secretions or to administer drug directly to the epithelial surface of the respiratory tract. With upper respiratory tract disease, a standard humidifier can be used; however, hydration of lower airway secretions requires use of an ultrasonic or compressed air nebulizer that will generate particles <4–5 μm in size. These are readily available through respiratory supply companies or via the Internet. Nebulization can be performed for 10–20 minutes as tolerated by the animal.

When nebulization is used to administer medication, a facemask should be used to provide direct delivery. Not all liquid preparations will physically form into micelles that can be distributed via nebulization. Some antibiotics (primarily aminoglycosides) can be nebulized and these are generally indicated for treatment of surface infection with *Bordetella bronchiseptica*. Albuterol, a beta-agonist bronchodilator can be nebulized. Budesonide is a steroid that can be nebulized but it requires use of a compressed-air nebulizer rather than an ultrasonic nebulizer. *N*-acetylcysteine, a mucolytic agent, is available in a form designed for nebulization; however, it may trigger bronchoconstriction when administered this way and can be somewhat toxic to airway epithelium.

Nebulization can also be used simply to hydrate airway secretions and facilitate removal from the lower airway. This can be very beneficial for animals that suffer from diseases resulting in excessive mucus production or pooling of secretions in the lower airways.

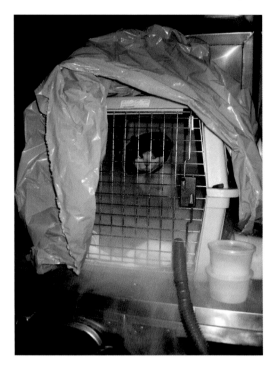

Figure 3.1.   Nebulization is performed in a cat carrier covered in plastic by using an ultrasonic nebulizer that creates particles <5 μm in size.

Sterile 0.9% saline dispensed as single-use vials without addition of preservatives is used most commonly, although some nebulizers require sterile water. A small aquarium, animal carrier, or plastic container can be modified to allow introduction of the nebulized liquid and venting of exhaled carbon dioxide (Figure 3.1). One to four treatments per day can be administered as needed. Gentle exercise or coupage following nebulization will encourage evacuation of airway mucus when treating lower respiratory disease (Figure 3.2).

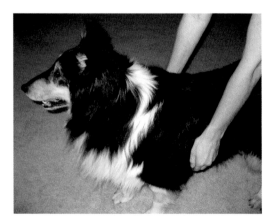

Figure 3.2.   Chest coupage is performed after nebulization by using cupped hands to percuss the chest in a ventral to dorsal and caudal to cranial manner.

Metered-Dose Inhalers

Various corticosteroid preparations are available as metered-dose inhalers (MDIs). Because animals will not actively inspire on command, administration of inhaled medication requires attachment of the MDI to a spacer device with facemask. Spacers are available from many respiratory supply companies including Respironics (Aerochamber®, Murrysville Pennsylvania, USA) and Trudell Medical (Aerokat®, Aerodawg®, London, Ontario, Canada; www.trudellmed.com). The spacer device collects the aerosolized drug generated by the MDI, and tidal respiration carries the particles into the lower airways. Investigation of pulmonary deposition of drug delivery with a MDI has not been performed, although in healthy cats, nebulization of a radiolabeled product administered via spacer and facemask resulted in adequate pulmonary deposition (Schulman et al. 2004). Clinically, this method of drug administration has proven efficacious in controlling clinical signs (Bexfield et al. 2006). A tightly fitting but comfortable facemask is critical for successful therapy, and it is important to ensure that the animal breathes normally for 8–10 seconds. Brachycephalic dogs often can be fit with a facemask designed for a cat or one obtained from a local pharmacy or respiratory supply company because the shape of the face is fairly similar to humans. For dolicocephalic breeds, anesthetic or cone-shaped facemasks may be required.

In dogs or cats with moderate-to-severe clinical manifestations of disease, standard doses of oral steroids are generally recommended during the first several weeks of inhaled therapy because of a delay in the efficacy of inhaled medications. The oral dose can be tapered downward depending on clinical response.

The most commonly recommended steroid is Flovent® (Fluticasone propionate inhalation powder), which is available in an MDI containing 120 doses to deliver 44, 110, or 220 μg/puff. Each dose can ameliorate experimentally induced airway eosinophilia in cats, (Cohn et al. 2010); however, the appropriate dose to use in naturally occurring disease is unknown. The MDI must be shaken well prior to actuation and should be attached to the spacer before the dose is ejected. Side effects of therapy have not been noted in veterinary patients to date. Clinical adrenal suppression can occur with long-term and high-dose use in humans, and although suppression of the hypothalamic–pituitary–adrenocortical axis does occur, systemic side effects are not noted in veterinary patients (Reinero et al. 2006, Cohn et al. 2008).

Inhaled medications are more expensive than oral medications, but they may result in improved owner compliance, particularly when animals are difficult to medicate orally and chronic therapy is required. In dogs, this method of therapy is particularly advantageous when side effects of steroids are severe or when concurrent diseases (diabetes, heart disease, pancreatitis, or renal disease) make oral steroid therapy undesirable. Many owners find that animals tolerate inhalation treatment readily, although problems may be encountered. Some cats are frightened by actuation of the MDI, although they can become habituated to the sound with training. The cat that suffers from acute asthmatic attacks may not tolerate application of the facemask and alternate therapy should be considered. An additional concern might be the competence of drug delivery because owners lack the ability to deploy the devise correctly, or because of a failure of the device to induce deposition of aerosol into constricted or mucus-laden airways. It is unclear whether this is a concern in veterinary patients. Finally, breath holding by the dog or cat can be a reason for treatment failure, although the newest spacing chamber created by Trudell Medical has a Flow-Vu indicator that allows visualization of respiratory movements at the valve of the chamber.

Adjunct Therapy

Oxygen Therapy

Supplemental oxygen should be provided to any animal presenting with respiratory difficulty as indicated by tachypnea, hyperpnea, cyanosis, or collapse, although it is important to realize that upper airway obstructive disease and pleural diseases are poorly responsive to oxygen administration alone. In those situations, alleviation of the obstruction and removal of pleural fluid or air to allow lung expansion are of critical importance. Oxygen can be supplied rapidly by attaching a facemask to an oxygen line and providing a high flow rate of oxygen directly to the patient. The disadvantage of this system is the need for continual patient restraint. An oxygen cage is generally less stressful to the patient and provides stable oxygen flow rates; however, examination of the animal is hindered. Nasal oxygen administration is suitable for animals that are able to breathe through the nose, and this method allows easy access for repeat examination and greater freedom of movement for the animal. To provide nasal oxygen, the outer surface of a red rubber tube is lightly coated with anesthetic gel and directed into the ventral nasal meatus. Tubes are advanced into the caudal aspect of the nasal cavity (approximately to the level of the medial canthus of the eye) to supply oxygen to the pharyngeal region and are glued or sutured in place (Figure 3.3). Oxygen flow rates of 1–5 liters/minute can provide 30–50% fraction inspired oxygen depending upon the size of the dog. Finally, an emergency oxygen tent can be created by inserting an oxygen supply tube into an Elizabethan collar covered with plastic wrap. An exhaust vent should be provided for the exit of carbon dioxide.

Oxygen supplementation at home can be helpful in dogs or cats with severe interstitial lung disease, particularly when the condition is complicated by pulmonary hypertension.

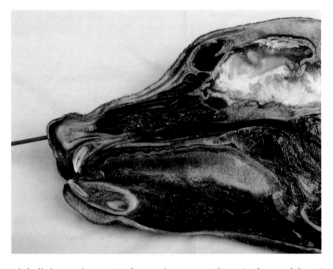

Figure 3.3. Transected skull shows placement of a nasal oxygen catheter in the caudal portion of the nasal cavity just rostral to the soft palate.

This type of therapy obviously requires a very dedicated owner and benefits are not easily quantifiable, although nightly administration can improve daytime activity in some animals. An oxygen chamber can be constructed from plexiglass or from an aquarium and must contain inlet and outlet valves. Oxygen is provided through a tank or compressor-driven system and the outlet allows egress of carbon dioxide. The fraction of inspired oxygen can often be maintained around 40–50% to provide an oxygen-enriched environment.

The level and extent of oxygen supplementation that can be supplied to a given animal without risking oxygen toxicity must be considered. Generally, moderate levels of oxygen (40–60%) can be administered for 24–48 hours without risking toxicity; however, the underlying disease process alters susceptibility to oxygen toxicity. Animals with aspiration lung injury, which generates both inflammatory and oxidative damage, are likely more susceptible to oxygen toxicity.

Animals with hypoxemia that are refractory to supplemental oxygen or those with excessive work of breathing resulting in respiratory muscle fatigue, require ventilatory support until lung disease or hypoventilation is adequately treated. Excessive respiratory muscle action during breathing or development of hyperthermia associated with the metabolic cost of breathing is indication for mechanical ventilation. Objective indicators for the need to provide mechanical ventilation are obtained from arterial blood gas values. An elevated P_aCO_2 (normal <45 mm Hg) indicates hypoventilation, and values that continue to increase over time (above 60 mmHg) generally require intervention. When a rising P_aCO_2 or when low P_aO_2 (<60 mm Hg, or pulse oximetry reading consistently <91%) fails to respond to supplemental oxygen therapy, mechanical ventilation should be considered. Because this requires constant monitoring, and is both labor intensive and technically challenging, referral to a critical care specialist is usually required.

Nutritional Therapy

Obesity is a common finding in the pet population and animals with chronic respiratory disease suffer from worsening of cough and respiratory effort when obesity results in poor lung expansion, reduced thoracic volume, or increased work of breathing. Obesity worsens clinical signs in dogs with chronic bronchitis by decreasing thoracic wall compliance and increasing abdominal pressure on the diaphragm. Improvements in exercise tolerance and arterial oxygenation can be seen with weight loss alone.

Owners should be given reasonable goals for an animal's optimal weight and the time in which weight loss can be achieved. A 1–2% weight loss per week is desirable but highly difficult to achieve (German et al. 2007). Marked energy restriction and rigorous owner cooperation is required. Close monitoring of owner compliance and using positive reinforcement seem to enhance the overall success. Animals can be started on 80% of their previous caloric intake. Alternately, the resting energy requirement (RER in kcal/day) can be used to calculate the daily calories to provide an obese animal to start a weight loss program: RER = 70 × (body weight in kg)$^{0.75}$. Use of a high-fiber, high-protein diet may improve participation in a weight loss program by enhancing satiety in patients and thus reducing food-seeking behavior (Weber et al. 2007). It is unclear whether the use of a commercially available appetite suppressants results in sustained weight control. When possible, the animal should be encouraged to participate in gradually increasing amounts of exercise.

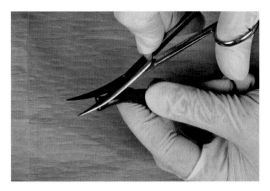

Figure 3.4. For removal of viscid pleural fluid associated with pyothorax, additional side holes can be cut in a red rubber catheter. Caution is warranted to avoid weakening the catheter with holes that are too large or placed too close together.

Chest Tube Placement

A chest tube is required for treatment of tension pneumothorax and pyothorax. It may occasionally be used to drain a large volume effusion from the pleural space. When placing a chest tube, sterile technique should be used and all necessary tools should be collected prior to initiation of the procedure. Commercially available chest tubes are supplied with a rigid, sharp stylet. Alternatively, a sterile red rubber catheter (18 French) with a 10-French urinary catheter inserted for support can be used. If a viscous pleural fluid is present, additional side holes should be made in the chest tube to limit clogging of the opening with fibrinous material (Figure 3.4). The animal is usually placed in lateral recumbency. Sedation is employed, but debilitated animals may not be able to tolerate excess anesthesia. The side of the thorax is liberally clipped for surgical preparation. Prior to inserting the chest tube, the desired position of the tube within the thorax should be visualized (Figure 3.5). Ideally,

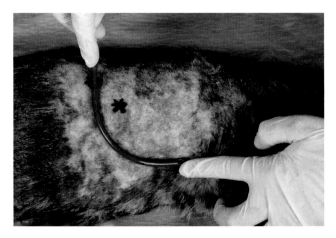

Figure 3.5. The chest tube should be placed through the skin at the tenth intercostal space and through the thorax at the eighth intercostal space. Ideally, it should lie on the ventral portion of the thorax. Any additional side holes made in the tube must be within the thoracic cavity.

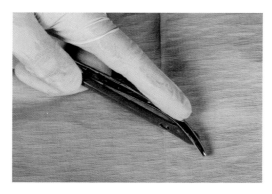

Figure 3.6. The red rubber catheter and stabilizing catheter are assembled and just the red rubber catheter is grasped with large curved hemostats. Approximately 1–2 cm of the instrument should precede the red rubber catheter into the chest cavity.

the chest tube will enter the skin at approximately the tenth intercostal space and will enter the thorax at a more ventral position at the eighth intercostal space. The chest tube will be directed ventrally to provide optimal drainage of fluid, and it should lie just ventral to the heart. Ensure that any side holes in the chest tube will lie within the thoracic cavity.

The site of the skin incision at the 10th intercostal space is infiltrated with local anesthesia (0.2–0.5 mL of lidocaine). An area ventral and cranial to the skin incision is chosen for entry of the chest tube into the thorax at the 8th intercostal space. This site should also be infiltrated with lidocaine down to the level of the pleura. Recall that the intercostal vessels and nerves lie on the caudal border of the rib. Thus, the tube should be inserted close to the cranial rib border to avoid trauma to these structures. After local anesthesia is instilled, the sterile surgical preparation is completed.

A stab incision is made at the caudal site on the thorax to allow easy entry of the chest tube through the skin. This incision should not be large since it must be sutured closed with a purse string pattern at the end of the procedure. Long curved forceps are used to grasp the chest tube, ensuring that that the supporting catheter is not trapped by the forceps. The sharp ends of the forceps will precede entry of the tube through the ribs (Figure 3.6). The chest tube is inserted through the skin and directed cranially and ventrally to create a subcutaneous tunnel at least two-rib spaces in length (Figure 3.7). The skin can be retracted

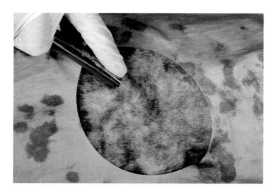

Figure 3.7. Hemostats are inserted through the skin and tunneled forward two-rib spaces.

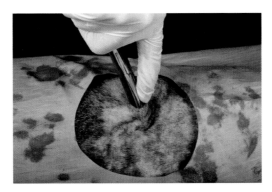

Figure 3.8. The curved hemostats are oriented perpendicular to the body wall to insert the red rubber catheter through the chest wall.

cranially, and this will assist in creating a subcutaneous tunnel that will act as a seal against air and bacteria entering the chest cavity. When the chest tube is in position to insert, it is raised to a 90° angle with the thorax (Figure 3.8). The grasp on the forceps should be maintained approximately 2–3 cm from the tip to limit entry of the instrument into the pleural cavity and prevent excessive penetration of the thorax. Controlled downward force is used to thrust the tube rapidly through the rib space.

After the tube is advanced into position in the ventral aspect of the chest cavity, the stylet is withdrawn and the end of the tube is quickly clamped with a large hemostat to prevent entrance of air into the chest. A purse string suture is used to close the skin incision. The distal end of the tube can be secured to the lateral aspect of the chest by using a "Chinese finger cot" suture (Figure 3.9). This will prevent the tube from being pulled out of the thorax if traction is applied to the tube.

When the tube has been sutured firmly in place, extension tubing with three-way stopcock and syringe are attached to the chest tube to insure a tight seal against leakage. The plastic flange on the extension set should be engaged in the closed position, the three-way stopcock (between the extension set and the syringe) is turned off to the patient, and a syringe completes the air seal. Gauze sponges loaded with antiseptic ointment are applied to the site on the chest where the tube exits the body and the tube is bandaged in place.

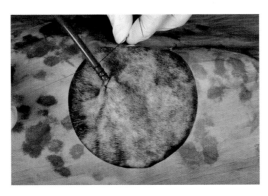

Figure 3.9. A purse string suture and finger cot pattern are used to close the incision and secure the chest tube in place.

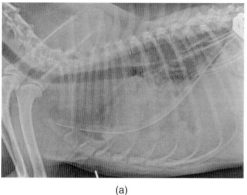
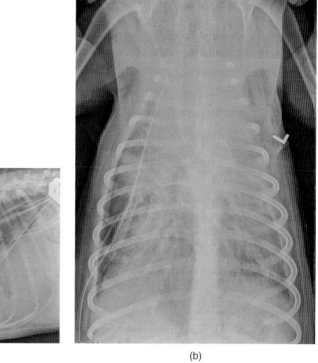

(a)   (b)

Figure 3.10. Left lateral (a) and dorsoventral (b) radiographs in a dog, showing proper placement of a chest tube for treatment of pyothorax. (Courtesy of Dr. Jason King, University of California, Davis.)

After placement of the chest tube, radiographs are performed to assess position of the tube (Figure 3.10). If a significant fluid volume is still present within the pleural space, placement of a second tube should be considered.

The chest is evacuated through continuous suction, whenever the animal exhibits respiratory distress, or on a predetermined schedule. Volume should be recorded to assess the production of air or fluid and to determine when the chest tube can be removed.

References

Bach JE, Kukanich B, Papich MG, et al. Evaluation of the bioavailability and pharmacokinetics of two extended-release theophylline formulations in dogs. J Am Vet Med Assoc. 2004; 224: 1113–1119.

Bexfield NH, Foale RD, Davison LJ, et al. Management of 13 cases of canine respiratory disease using inhaled corticosteroids. J Small Anim Pract. 2006; 47: 377–382.

Cohn LA, DeClue AE, Cohen RL, Reinero CL. Effects of fluticasone propionate dose in an experimental model of feline asthma J Fel Med Surg. 2010; 12: 91–96.

Cohn LA, DeClue AE, Reinero CR. Endocrine and immunologic effects of inhaled fluticasone propionate in healthy dogs. J Vet Int Med. 2008; 22: 37–43.

Dossin O, Grue P, Thomas E. Comparative field evaluation of marbofloxacin tablets in the treatment of feline upper respiratory tract infections. J Small An Pract. 1998; 39: 286–289.

Dye JA, McKiernan BC, Rozanski EA, et al. Bronchopulmonary disease in the cat: historical, physical, radiographic, clinicopathologic, and pulmonary functional evaluation of 24 affected and 15 healthy cats. J Vet Int Med. 1996; 10, 385–400.

German AJ, Holden SL, Bissot T, et al. Dietary energy restriction and successful weight loss in obese client-owned dogs. J Vet Int Med. 2007; 21: 1174–1180.

Guenther-Yenke CL, McKiernan BC, Papich MG, et al. Pharmacokinetics of an extended-release theophylline product in cats. J Am Vet Med Assoc. 2007; 231: 900–906.

Hunter RP, Lunch MJ, Ericson JF, et al. Pharmacokinetics, oral bioavailability, and tissue distribution of azithromycin in cats. J Vet Pharmacol Ther. 1995; 18: 38–46.

Intorre L, Mengozzi G, Maccheroni M, et al. Enrofloxacin–theophylline interaction: Influence of enrofloxacin on theophylline steady-state pharmacokinetics in the Beagle dog. J Vet Pharmacol Ther. 1995; 18: 352–356.

Jang SS, Breher JE, Dabaco LA, et al. Organisms isolated from dogs and cats with anaerobic infections and susceptibility to selected antimicrobial agents. J Am Vet Med Assoc. 1997; 210: 1610–1614.

Johnson LR, Foley JE, De Cock HEV, et al. Assessment of infectious organisms associated with chronic rhinosinusitis in cats. J Am Vet Med Assoc. 2005; 227: 579–585.

Padrid PA, Hornof W, Kurpershoek C, et al. Canine chronic bronchitis: A pathophysiologic evaluation of 18 cases. J Vet Int Med. 1990; 4: 172–181.

Reinero CR, Brownlee L, Decile KC, et al. Inhaled flunisolide suppresses the hypothalamic–pituitary–adrenocortical axis, but has minimal systemic immune effects in healthy cats. J Vet Int Med. 2006; 20: 57–64.

Reinero CR, Delgado C, Spinka C, et al. Enantiomer-specific effects of albuterol on airway inflammation in healthy and asthmatic cats. Int Arch Allergy Immunol. 2009; 150: 43–50.

Schulman RL, Crochik SS, Kneller SJ, et al. Investigation of pulmonary deposition of a nebulized radiopharmaceutical agent in awake cats. Am J Vet Res. 2004; 65: 806–809.

Weber M, Bissot T, Servet E, et al. A high-protein, high-fiber diet designed for weight loss improves satiety in dogs. J Vet Int Med. 2007; 21: 1203–1208.

Windsor RC, Johnson LR, Herrgesell EJ, De Cock HEV. Lymphoplasmacytic rhinitis in 37 dogs: 1997–2002. J Am Vet Med Assoc. 2004; 224: 1952–1957.

Nasal Disorders 4

Structural Diseases

Stenotic Nares and Brachycephalic Syndrome

Pathophysiology

Brachycephalic airway syndrome (BAS) is a congenital disorder resulting from primary conformational defects (stenotic nares or an elongated soft palate), which obstruct flow of air through the upper airways. Increased flow and pressure effects on the soft tissue structures of the larynx result in inflammation that leads to secondary findings of everted laryngeal saccules, thickening of the soft palate, and in the final stages, laryngeal collapse. In the bulldog, tracheal hypoplasia may be encountered as an additional component of BAS. BAS results from shortening of the nasal cavity and in some dogs (particularly Pugs) it can be accompanied by caudal protrusion of nasal turbinates into the nasopharynx (Figure 4.1), resulting in further obstruction of nasal airflow (Ginn et al. 2008).

History and signalment

Brachycephalic syndrome is common in bulldogs (English and French), Pugs, and Boston Terriers, and is also seen in Himalayan and Persian cats (Figure 4.2). Clinical signs include stertor, snoring or snuffling, gagging, exercise intolerance, respiratory difficulty, and collapse. Some dogs (particularly bulldogs) have vomiting or regurgitation due to concurrent gastroesophageal disease caused by reflux, inflammation, or an esophageal diverticulum (Poncet et al. 2005). Animals can be very young or aged (6 weeks to 14 years of age) when clinical signs require evaluation and correction.

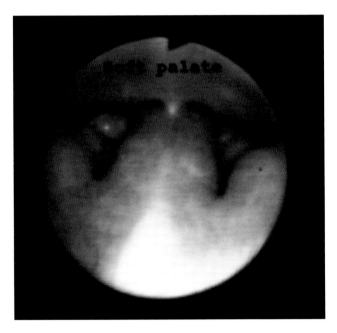

Figure 4.1. Retroflex view of the choanae in a pug shows hyperemic and swollen turbinates that are bulging into the nasopharynx and contributing to upper airway obstruction.

Physical examination

Stenotic nares can be visualized on physical examination and must be compared to breed standards. Audible stertor is due to turbulent airflow through the nasal cavity, past everted saccules, or past an elongated soft palate. Stertor is often evident on inspiration and expiration. If laryngeal collapse is presence, stridor may be detected on inspiration with auscultation of the larynx. In dogs with tracheal hypoplasia, high-pitched inspiratory wheezes

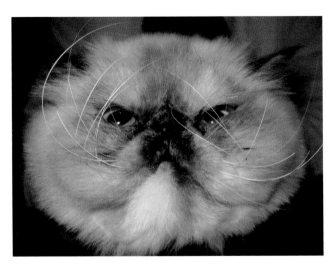

Figure 4.2. Stenotic nares in a brachycephalic cat.

can sometimes be auscultated over the trachea. The remainder of the physical examination is usually within normal limits, although obesity often worsens the clinical presentation.

Diagnostic findings

Cervical and thoracic radiographs are useful for subjective evaluation of the length and thickness of the soft palate and to assess tracheal size when tracheal hypoplasia is suspected. Two methods have been reported to evaluate tracheal size. One compares tracheal lumen diameter in the thoracic region to the third rib. A normal dimension is >3.0 (Suter 1984). In the second method, tracheal lumen diameter at the thoracic inlet is compared to the height of the thoracic inlet. The normal ratio in the bulldog is >0.127, in the non-bulldog brachycephalic is >0.160, and in the normal dog is >0.204 (Harvey and Fink 1982).

Documentation of soft palate elongation and assessment of laryngeal structures requires sedation for direct visualization, and because of anesthetic concerns with brachycephalic breeds, surgical correction should be planned at the time the diagnosis is confirmed. Normally, the soft palate should extend only 1–2 mm caudal to the tip of the epiglottis. In some cases, rostral retraction of the soft palate is required to assess the extent of elongation. Eversion of laryngeal saccules can be visualized as rounded and bulging soft tissue structures emerging from the ventral portion of the laryngeal aditus, just lateral to the vocal folds (Figure 4.3). Laryngeal collapse can be recognized as medial displacement of the arytenoid cartilages, possibly due to chronic weakening of the laryngeal abductor muscles or to some degree of chondromalacia (Figure 4.3). This condition must be distinguished from laryngeal paralysis, a disorder in which arytenoid cartilages do not abduct on inspiration but are normally positioned. Laryngeal collapse is designated grade 2 when the cuneiform processes are involved and grade 3 when the corniculate processes are collapsed. (Eversion of the laryngeal saccules is sometimes referred to as grade 1 laryngeal collapse.) If a flexible

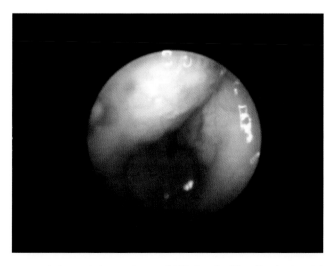

Figure 4.3. This laryngoscopic image is from a 9-year-old FS Cavalier King Charles Spaniel presented for chronic panting and syncope. Everted and edematous laryngeal saccules are evident ventrally in the image. Dorsal to the laryngeal aditus, the corniculate processes of the arytenoid are folding across midline, indicative of grade 3 laryngeal collapse.

endoscope is available, a retroflex examination of the nasopharynx should be performed to document the presence of nasopharyngeal turbinates as these can lead to continued obstructed breathing following surgical correction of other lesions.

Treatment

Weight reduction is essential to reduce the work of breathing in animals with brachycephalic syndrome, and when possible, this should be achieved prior to surgery to reduce complications associated with anesthesia. Stenotic nares and elongated soft palate are amenable to surgical resection with a scalpel or CO_2 laser via wedge resection and staphylectomy, respectively. Excessive shortening of the soft palate is generally not recommended because this can result in nasal regurgitation, although some surgeons believe it is an appropriate technique. In some cases, saccular eversion will resolve when airflow has improved; however, in some dogs, chronic protrusion of the saccules results in irreversible hyperplasia that requires resection. Some surgeons elect to remove a single saccule initially to avoid mucosal apposition during the healing phase that could result in laryngeal stenosis. Others remove both saccules and place a temporary tracheostomy tube in case upper airway swelling results in obstruction. Currently, no specific treatment is available for laryngeal collapse, and the success of unilateral lateralization is relatively low. For dogs with severe stridor or respiratory distress, a permanent tracheostomy should be considered if weight loss and surgical correction of other lesions fail to alleviate respiratory difficulty. More aggressive therapy for brachycephalic syndrome includes laser resection of internal nasal turbinates.

The age at which this surgery should optimally be performed is unknown; however, it would seem wise to correct conformational disorders early in life to prevent development of secondary obstructive disease.

Prognosis

Surgical resection of upper airway obstruction is associated with an excellent outcome in the vast majority of cases. Perioperative mortality is low and postoperative complications of regurgitation or nasal discharge are generally mild. Dehiscence of the palatal repair is the most serious event encountered but occurs rarely. Animals that have concurrent gastroesophageal signs often have resolution or abolition of gastrointestinal signs following surgery (Poncet et al. 2006), although some may require continual use of prokinetic and acid reducing drugs.

Nasal Foreign Body

History and signalment

Foreign material can be aspirated directly into the nasal cavity through the nares or may lodge in the nasopharynx when the animal retches material from the oral cavity into the region above the palate. Animals with a nasal foreign body usually present with an acute onset of paroxysmal sneezing or reverse sneezing, nasal discharge, epistaxis, and pawing or rubbing at the face, although chronic signs can also be seen. Foreign bodies that are firmly lodged in the nasal cavity or in the nasopharynx can also result in chronic nasal discharge or halitosis.

Physical examination

Affected animals usually display unilateral mucopurulent or serosanguineous nasal discharge, and nasal airflow is preserved. In chronic cases, or if secondary nasal aspergillosis results, regional lymph node enlargement can be found.

Diagnosis and treatment

Animals are fully anesthetized for evaluation of the nasal cavity. Radiographs are usually recommended prior to examination of the nasal cavity to help guide removal of a radiodense foreign body; however, organic objects are usually not visible radiographically. In more chronic cases, secondary changes of increased fluid density or bony lysis can help locate the site of the foreign material.

Whenever possible, the caudal nasopharynx should be examined for a foreign body as well as both nasal cavities. If a flexible endoscope is not available, copious antegrade and retrograde flush of the nasal cavity can dislodge a foreign body (see Chapter 2). If the nasal cavity cannot be fully visualized with available equipment, gentle probing and retraction of alligator forceps can be successful in retrieving a foreign body. In rare instances an exploratory rhinotomy may be required. This is most likely when a large smooth foreign body (such as a stone) cannot be removed endoscopically. After foreign body retrieval, a broad-spectrum antibiotic is usually administered for 7 days to treat secondary infection.

Prognosis

In some cases, a foreign body can cause permanent damage to the nasal structures that allows development of secondary fungal rhinitis or results in chronic nasal discharge associated with alterations in turbinates and mucus production. In these cases, intermittent antibiotic therapy may be required to control clinical signs.

Tooth Root Abscess or Oronasal Fistula

History and signalment

Dental-related nasal disease usually affects the carnassial or canine tooth in older animals and results in unilateral mucopurulent to hemorrhagic nasal discharge. The animal may display difficulty or pain while eating or opening the mouth. Anorexia, drooling, and halitosis can be reported.

Physical examination

Unilateral nasal discharge should raise the suspicion of dental-related disease; however, it is important to note that the dental or gingival disease may not be obvious without an examination under anesthesia. Nasal airflow is preserved in animals with dental-related nasal disease. Oral or facial pain or swelling and regional lymphadenopathy can be found in some cases. With a carnassial tooth abscess, an expanding facial swelling may develop immediately below the eye on the affected side.

Diagnostic findings

Skull or dental radiographs highlighting the affected area can reveal bony loss surrounding a tooth root or a retained tooth root. In cases with chronic dental disease, destruction of turbinates can be seen on radiographs, computed tomography (CT), or rhinoscopy. Use of a periodontal probe to detect deep (>1 mm in the cat and >1–3 mm in the dog) periodontal pockets can identify occult tooth root disease.

Treatment

Effective treatment requires removal of the tooth and all roots. In some instances, bony curettage may be required or surgical debridement and closure of a fistula. A 7–10-day course of antibiotics (with a potentiated penicillin or clindamycin) is often used to treat secondary infection.

Prognosis

Generally nasal discharge resolves with tooth removal; however, as with a foreign body, alterations in turbinate structures can result in continued mucus production. Sequestration of a tooth root or a devitalized bony fragment must be ruled out in such cases.

Nasopharyngeal Stenosis

Pathophysiology

The opening to the caudal nasopharynx in dogs and cats is normally 1–2 cm across and can be greatly reduced or obliterated by a web of scar tissue. Nasopharyngeal stenosis (NPS) is thought to occur either as a congenital lesion in which the caudal opening of the choanae is malformed, or as an acquired lesion resulting from chronic inflammation in the caudal aspect of the nasal cavity that forms a cicatrix. Inflammation may result from chronic upper respiratory tract disease or from regurgitation of esophageal or gastric contents into the nasopharynx. The scar may be unilateral or extend across the entire choanae (Figure 4.4).

History and signalment

The predominant clinical feature of this disorder is obstruction of airflow through the nasal cavity. Stertorous respiration or snoring sounds are commonly reported. In some cases, this condition is preceded or accompanied by nasal discharge. When the deformation or scar is bilateral or circumferential, the animal will display mouth breathing because of an inability to breathe through the nose. It is usually nonprogressive and not associated with systemic disease, although inappetance has been reported in some cats.

Physical examination

The primary recognizable exam feature is a loud upper respiratory noise that may be stertorous (snoring) or stridorous. Respiratory difficulty is present on inspiration and there is a lack of nasal airflow that depends on the degree of stenosis. Respiratory distress occurs when the mouth is closed and nasal breathing is required.

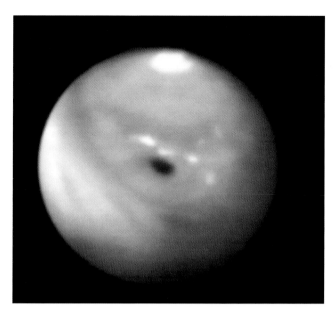

Figure 4.4. Retroflex view of the choanae in a 17-year-old FS DSH presented for an 8-year history of difficulty breathing. In this case, stenosis of the nasopharynx reduces the diameter to less than a millimeter.

Diagnostic findings

Primary differential diagnoses include nasal obstruction due to neoplasia, a nasopharyngeal polyp, cryptococcosis (in the dog or cat), or aspergillosis (in the cat). NPS is most easily diagnosed using a flexible endoscope to obtain a view of the nasopharynx. Alternately, the obstruction can be appreciated by passing a 3–8-French catheter caudally through the ventral meatus into the oropharyngeal region. In the normal animal, this should pass easily into the pharynx; however, a stenosed region will block passage of the catheter. Tissue malformation in the choanal region can often be visualized on CT with sagittal reconstruction of the image.

Treatment

Treatment of this obstructive breathing disorder can be achieved by balloon dilation of the region under fluoroscopy or endoscopy, although several episodes may be required. Stent placement has also been successful in alleviating the obstruction (Berent et al. 2008). The membrane is too thick to be broken down manually or with a standard catheter. If surgery is contemplated, the approach to the caudal nasopharynx is through a midline incision in the soft palate. Iris scissors can be used to excise the nasopharyngeal membrane.

Prognosis

NPS represents a benign lesion; however, some owners report loss of appetite or lethargy related to nasal obstruction. In cats with concurrent rhinitis, it is unclear whether the presence of stenosis impacts clinical response to therapy.

Infectious Diseases

Acute Feline Upper Respiratory Tract Disease

Pathophysiology

The organisms most commonly implicated in infectious upper respiratory tract disease in kittens include feline herpes-virus 1 (FHV-1), feline calicivirus (FCV), *Chlamydophila felis*, *Mycoplasma*, and *Bordetella*. Other viruses may also be involved. Infection occurs via inhalation or via contact with mucosal membranes of the nose or ocular surface. Viral infection of the epithelial cells results in cell death and predisposes the respiratory tract to bacterial infection. However, the bacteria involved can also act as primary respiratory pathogens, and infection with bacteria alone can result in substantial clinical disease. *Chlamydophila felis* results in systemic infection although clinical signs may be manifest in the conjunctiva alone.

Viral infection is usually self-limiting with resolution of disease within 7–10 days. Viral shedding occurs within 1–3 days of infection and persists for up to 3 weeks, providing a constant source of virus in the environment. Both FHV-1 and FCV persist in the cat population as a carrier state and viral shedding can be reactivated during stressful periods. A virulent form of FCV has been associated with outbreaks of ulcerative lesions around the face, facial and forelimb edema, and fatal pneumonia with mortality rates of ~40% (Hurley et al. 2004).

History and signalment

Young kittens (2 weeks to 4 months old) are affected most commonly although older kittens and cats can develop signs of acute upper respiratory tract disease when exposed to high concentrations of pathogens in a shelter environment. Older cats are more severely affected by the virulent form of FCV, and any age cat may develop *Chlamydophila* conjunctivitis.

Physical examination

Sneezing and serous to mucoid oculo-nasal discharge are the classic findings in acute feline upper respiratory tract disease (FURTD). Fever and systemic signs of illness (lethargy and anorexia) are commonly seen. FHV-1 has a predilection for ocular infection, and conjunctival hyperemia and corneal disease are common. Tracheitis is also reported secondary to FHV-1 infection but signs are rarely observed clinically. FCV can cause lingual ulcers and pneumonia, while *Chlamydophila* is most likely to cause severe chemosis, which can be unilateral or bilateral.

Diagnostic findings

In general, FURTD is a clinical diagnosis. Testing is available through culture or polymerase chain reaction for FHV-1; however, the presence of virus does not correlate with disease (Maggs et al. 1999). The presence of FCV can be confirmed through virus isolation or reverse transcriptase PCR for the RNA virus, although positive tests are expected in chronic shedders, making it difficult to correlate the test result with disease activity. The virulent form of FCV is diagnosed based on clinical signs and physical examination.

Bacterial culture may be helpful in determining appropriate antibiotic therapy for *Mycoplasma* or *Bordetella*; however, this is rarely performed in the setting of acute upper respiratory tract disease. Diagnostic tests including virus isolation, bacterial culture, and PCR should be used in disease outbreaks that are associated with high morbidity or mortality to identify potential infecting organisms and institute appropriate control measures. These tests have also proven useful in providing details on the spread of organisms within confined populations. In a shelter study, shedding of FHV-1 was shown to increase from 4 to 52% after 1 week (Pedersen et al. 2004).

Treatment

Supportive care will aid in resolution of signs related to viral infection. The eyes and nose should be kept clear of exudate, hydration and adequate nutrition should be ensured, and animals should be kept in a warm environment. Steam inhalation to humidify inhaled air and use of lubricating eye ointment to manage virally mediated keratoconjunctivitis sicca can also improve overall health. Systemic antibiotic therapy is directed at control of secondary bacterial infection, and most antibiotics are efficacious, including amoxicillin–clavulanate and pradofloxacin, although if infection by *Mycoplasma* is documented, a quinolone or tetracycline drug would be recommended. Treatment of *Chlamydophila* requires at 4–6 weeks of therapy with doxycycline at 10 mg/kg/day.

Lysine has been recommended to reduce viral replication and decrease clinical signs associated with FHV-1 infection. However, dietary supplementation did not prove efficacious in a natural disease setting, (Maggs et al. 2007) and bolus administration of 250–500 mg PO BID is required to reduce viral replication.

A novel antiviral therapy for FCV that blocks virus synthesis by molecular interference with the initiation of translation was recently shown to reduce the severity of oral ulcers and reduce FCV shedding in an outbreak situation (Smith et al. 2008). Treatment also reduced mortality in an outbreak of virulent FCV, suggesting that this therapy could show promise in management of severe viral disease.

Prognosis

Most kittens survive an episode of acute upper respiratory infection. It is unclear whether severe infection at an early age plays a role in development of chronic rhinosinusitis. When disease is observed in a shelter or cattery situation, implementation of control measures with improved hygiene is needed. FHV-1 is labile in the environment and is readily killed by bleach or detergent; however, FCV can persist for up to 1 month and is more resistant to standard cleaning methods. Aerosolization is the prime method of infection, and isolation of sneezing or coughing cats can help limit spread. However, fomites can also spread disease, and general infection control should be stressed. Vaccination against upper respiratory viruses (FHV-1 and FCV) reduces clinical signs and may help limit spread of disease.

Cryptococcosis

Pathophysiology

Cryptococcus is a dimorphic fungus that exists in the yeast form in the animal. Various species enjoy a specific geographic distribution with *Cryptococcus neoformans* var. *grubii* found in bird guano worldwide, *C. neoformans* var. *neoformans* found primarily in bird guano in Europe, and *Cryptococcus gattii* localized primarily in Eucalyptus trees in Australia and numerous trees in Vancouver, Canada. Disease is thought to be spread primarily through inhalation with initial infection in the nasal cavity and subsequent spread to the nasopharynx or central nervous system, although direct inoculation causing skin infection may also occur.

History and signalment

Cryptococcal infection has been reported in all ages of animals, although young adults appear to be affected most often. Disease is reported much more commonly in cats than in dogs, with Siamese and Abyssinian cats overrepresented. Respiratory complaints include facial distortion, sneezing, chronic mucopurulent nasal discharge, and stertor. Lower respiratory infection occurs much less commonly, but signs of pneumonia may be present. Nonrespiratory complaints include nonhealing craterous skin lesions, blindness due to retinal detachment or optic neuritis, and central nervous system signs such as circling, seizures, ataxia, or vestibular disease.

Physical examination

The classic finding for nasal cryptococcosis is firm swelling along the dorsum of the nose. It can be central or unilateral, at the bridge of the nose or on the tip. In some cases, a mass can be seen protruding from the nose (Figure 4.5). Regional lymphadenopathy is not uncommon. In cases with lower respiratory tract disease, tachypnea may be noted and abnormal lung sounds may be found because of lobar consolidation. In some animals, ulcerated and craterous skin lesions are evident. Every cat suspected of cryptococcosis should have a thorough fundic examination to look for chorioretinitis. This inflammatory condition of the choroid and retina can appear as a hyporeflective, round to geographic,

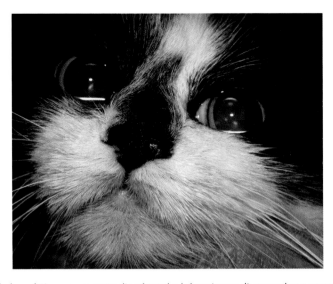

Figure 4.5. This fleshy soft tissue mass protruding from the left naris was diagnosed as a cryptococcal granuloma.

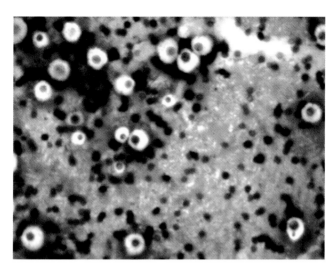

Figure 4.6. Cytology of an impression smear from a nasal mass in a cat. Wright's stain has been applied and reveals multiple 3–8 μm round organisms surrounded by a clear capsule ranging in size from 10 to 30 μm. Fungal culture was positive for *C. gattii*.

white to gray, sometimes raised fluffy lesion when active, or as a dark circular region on the retina when the lesion has scarred or healed.

Diagnostic findings

Diagnosis involves identification of a fungal organism (5–8 μm in size) with a clear polysaccharide coat (~30 μm in diameter) in cytology of exudate, aspirates, impression smears, or a squash preparation of a biopsy specimen (Figure 4.6). Wright's stain, Diff Quik, or iodine can be used. Because the fungal organism is so characteristic, cytologic examination of nasal smears from cats with chronic nasal discharge is warranted for quick differentiation of a fungal infection from other causes of nasal discharge, although nonencapsulated forms of *Cryptococcus* may confuse the diagnosis. Serology is recommended by using the latex capsular agglutination titer (LCAT), which offers a sensitive and specific method for diagnosis by detecting the cryptococcal antigen. A titer greater than 1:1 is positive, and the magnitude of the LCAT can be used to follow response to therapy.

Occasionally a fungal culture will be positive for *Cryptococcus* in the absence of clinical disease due to colonization of the nasal cavity without infection; however, in animals with signs consistent with disease, culture for cryptococcosis is recommended to determine the serotype of the organism involved. This will help establish the epidemiology of infection and can define the manifestations of disease and response to therapy for different strains. Depending on the clinical presentation and physical examination findings, chest radiographs or abdominal ultrasound should be performed to stage the disease. A complete blood count, chemistry profile, and urinalysis are performed to assess the general health of the animal and retroviral testing should be performed in the cat. Concurrent immunosuppressive disease due to FeLV may be associated with a worse prognosis for cure or control of disease, and FIV-infected cats may require longer duration of treatment.

Treatment

Cryptococcosis is typically treated with oral azole therapy, and prolonged therapy (4–12 months) should be anticipated (see Chapter 3). Itraconazole (50–100 mg/cat/day) is reportedly efficacious in approximately 50% cases of nasal cryptococcosis (Medleau et al. 1995) while fluconazole at a dose of 25–100 mg/cat PO BID resulted in cure of nasal cryptococcosis in 97% of cats, despite disseminated disease or concurrent FIV infection in up to 28% of cases (Malik et al. 1992). Duration of treatment required to achieve control of disease with fluconazole was significantly shorter than with itraconazole (4 versus 9 months) (O'Brien et al. 2006). Fluconazole is preferred if ocular involvement is documented because of better penetration of the blood ocular barrier, and if central nervous system involvement is suspected or confirmed based on physical examination, clinical signs, brain imaging, or CSF tap, fluconazole is used in combination with flucytosine because of improved efficacy in penetrating the blood–brain barrier. Posaconazole and voriconazole may also prove useful in management of cryptococcosis.

Terbinafine, a synthetic allylamine, can be employed in cats that do not respond appropriately to azole therapy or those that develop side effects while treated with azoles. It may be used alone or in combination with an azole.

Fungicidal treatment is needed in cases with severe cryptococcocis, and amphotericin B has proven effective in inducing remission. Subcutaneous administration of amphotericin B should be considered in animals that cannot tolerate oral medications. Nephrotoxicity is limited with this mode of administration, although cure of cryptococcosis can require a cumulative dose over 20 mg/kg (Malik et al. 1996).

Prognosis

The latex agglutination titer can be used to follow the course of disease and response to treatment. A twofold reduction in antigen titer per month is desired, although titers can be rechecked every 2–3 months rather than monthly. Treatment for cryptococcosis is continued until the latex agglutination titer to capsular antigen is >1:1. Cats with intranasal cryptococcosis have a slightly lower percentage of resolution of disease than those with cutaneous signs only, and central nervous system infection is the least responsive. Cats that fail to show a reduction in antigen titer over several months are less likely to achieve resolution of disease and may be resistant to the antifungal drug in use. In these cases, culture and susceptibility testing should be considered. Recurrence of cryptococcosis may occur months to years after apparent cure, and a relapse rate of 17% has been reported (O'Brien et al. 2006).

Canine Nasal Aspergillosis

Pathophysiology

Aspergillus is a branching septate mold that is ubiquitous in the environment. Nasal aspergillosis can result from infection with several different *Aspergillus* species, although infection with *Aspergillus fumigatus* is most common. Nasal aspergillosis occurs as a primary infection in healthy dogs, but the fungus can also colonize the nasal cavity and/or frontal sinuses following trauma, inhalation of a foreign body, or in conjunction with a neoplastic process. *Aspergillus* results in mucosal infection of the nasal cavity and/or sinuses with formation of fungal granulomas or plaque lesions. Toxins produced by the fungus and the local inflammatory response are likely responsible for the severe destruction and collapse of turbinates that occurs with infection. The nasal mucosa responds to infection by upregulation of proinflammatory cytokines (IL-6, IL-12, IL-18, and TNF-α) as well as the immunomodulatory cytokine IL-10, which may reduce tissue injury but also limit the host's ability to clear the organism from the nose (Peeters et al. 2006).

History and signalment

Nasal aspergillosis is most commonly encountered in young to middle-aged dolicocephalic dogs. Animals tend to have a long-standing history (4–6 months) of purulent or hemorrhagic nasal discharge and sneezing. Dogs may become head-shy or exhibit pain. Recognition of neurologic signs such as seizures or obtundation suggests fungal invasion of the central nervous system through the cribriform plate.

Physical examination

Nasal discharge is commonly unilateral but can become bilateral with time when disease erodes through the septum. Dogs typically have preservation of nasal airflow because of marked turbinate destruction. Depigmentation of the nares with or without ulceration is found in approximately 40% of canine cases. Some dogs display marked facial or skull pain on palpation. Ipsilateral lymphadenopathy is found occasionally due to a reactive lymph node response; however, affected animals remain systemically healthy.

Diagnostic findings

A minimum database is typically unremarkable but may show evidence of chronic infection, with neutrophilia, monocytosis, and hyperglobinemia. An agar gel immunodiffusion test (AGID) using an *Aspergillus* antigen prepared from cultures of *A. fumigatus*, *A. niger*, and *A. flavus* has proven useful in confirming the clinical suspicion of aspergillosis in dogs. Positive AGID for *Aspergillus* spp. was highly suggestive of nasal aspergillosis in one study, with a positive predictive value of 94%; however, false-negative results were found in almost one-third of cases (Pomrantz et al. 2007).

In a recent study on cytologic diagnosis of aspergillosis, direct smear of nasal discharge or swab revealed fungal hyphae in a minority (<20%) of cases (De Lorenzi et al. 2006). Cytology of a swab or biopsy sample collected endoscopically was more likely (>90%) to demonstrate fungal spores. A recent study on the utility of fungal cultures in the diagnosis of canine nasal aspergillosis reported moderate sensitivity (77%) but high specificity (100%) (Pomrantz et al. 2007). It is important to note that in that study, the material submitted for culture was from a visualized fungal plaque and therefore, a low number of false-positive values would be expected. Fungal culture of nasal discharge has been associated with much lower sensitivity and specificity and is not recommended.

More definitive diagnosis and disease staging is obtained by finding the characteristic imaging findings with radiography or CT scan and with rhinoscopic detection of plaque lesions. Skull radiographs show variable degrees of turbinate lysis (unilateral or bilateral) and increased radiolucency (Figure 4.7). The majority of dogs (75% or more) have sinus involvement, and a frontal view of the skull should be included in the radiographic examination to look for a fungal granuloma in the sinus (Figure 4.7). In some cases, this might

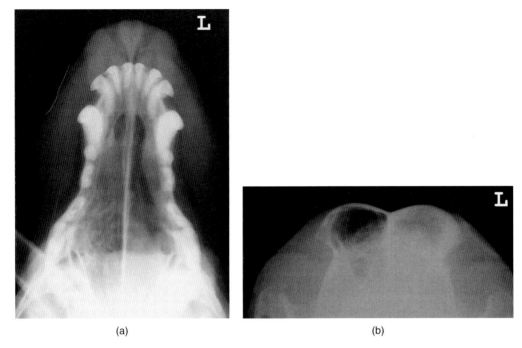

(a) (b)

Figure 4.7. Open mouth view (a) of the nasal cavity in a 2-year-old MC Golden Retriever presented for left-sided nasal discharge. Asymmetry is evident with lucency noted intranasally on the left side. An amorphous soft tissue density can be appreciated caudally. Turbinate structures on the right appear within normal limits. Frontal sinus image (b) of the same dog reveals a heterogeneous soft tissue density within the left frontal sinus. Sinuscopic examination and histopathology confirmed a fungal granuloma within the sinus.

be the only location in which the granuloma can be identified (Johnson et al. 2006). CT scan is preferred for evaluation of dogs suspected of nasal aspergillosis. CT scans typically reveal unilateral loss of turbinate structures and may show granulomatous fungal lesions, particularly in the frontal sinus (Figure 4.8). The integrity of the cribriform plate can also be assessed, which aids in making the decision to use topical antifungal therapy (Figure 4.8). Dogs with destruction of the cribriform plate are more susceptible to central nervous system complications from edema or inflammation that results from contact of the vehicle and antifungal medication with the meninges.

Rhinoscopic examination of the nasal cavity is remarkable for severe destruction of turbinates with increased space within the nasal cavity. Fungal plaques may be white, green, or black and are surrounded by granulomatous and hemorrhagic inflammation (Figure 4.9). It is critical to obtain a sample from the fungal plaque for cytologic, histopathologic, and mycologic evaluation (Figure 4.10). Definitive diagnosis of aspergillosis relies on a combination of radiographic evidence, rhinoscopic examination, cytologic or histopathologic changes, and serology.

Treatment

Nasal aspergillosis in the dog is best treated with local instillation of clotrimazole or enilconazole, with resolution reported in up to 67–85% of cases following multiple infusions

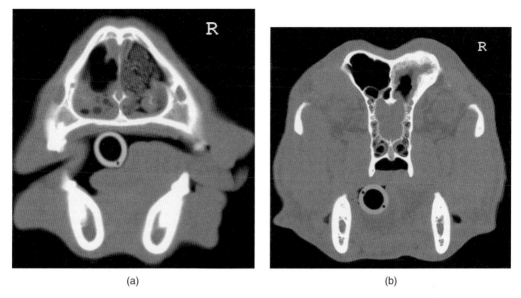

(a)   (b)

Figure 4.8.   CT images from two dogs with confirmed sinonasal aspergillosis. Rostrally (a), cavitation of the nasal cavity is noted on the left side with collapse of turbinates. In the region of the frontal sinus (b), hyperostosis of the right frontal sinus is noted along with an adherent soft tissue density surrounding the sinus. On the ventral floor of the frontal sinus, a breach in the cribriform plate is noted with local destruction by fungal infection.

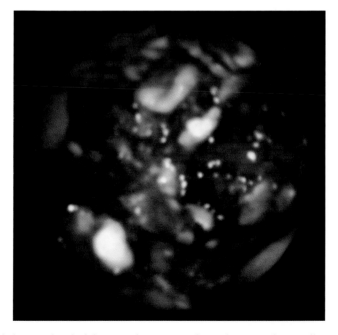

Figure 4.9.   Fungal plaques identified during endoscopy in a dog with sinonasal aspergillus.

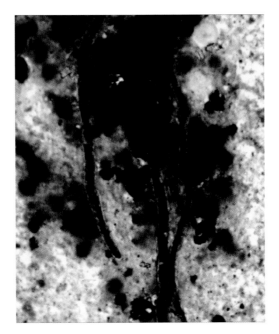

Figure 4.10.   New methylene blue staining of an impression smear from the sample visualized in Figure 4.9 reveals rectangular, septate hyphae and conidia consistent with *Aspergillus* spp.

(Zonderland et al. 2002, Pomrantz and Johnson in press). Fungal plaques must be meticulously debrided from the nasal cavity and frontal sinus. In many cases, sinus trephination, debridement, and local treatment are required (Johnson et al. 2006). Prior to infusion of antifungal medication, the nasopharynx is occluded with a 24-French Foley catheter, 10-French drug delivery catheters are placed in the nasal cavity, and the nares are blocked with 12-French Foley catheters to maintain the drug at the site of infection (Figure 4.11). The

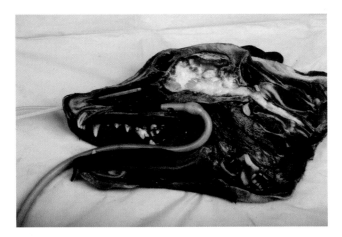

Figure 4.11.   Placement of nasal catheters for treatment of sinonasal aspergillosis. A 24-French Foley catheter is placed in the nasopharynx to prevent leakage of material into the oral cavity. Ten-French polypropylene catheters are used to deliver topical therapy, and 12-French Foley catheters are used to obstruct the nares and retain drug within the nasal cavity for the 1-hour infusion.

drug is instilled for 1 hour and the animal's head is rotated into dorsal, left lateral, right lateral, and dorsal recumbency every 15 minutes. This method provides treatment of both nasal cavities and both frontal sinuses as the solution drains down to fill the space.

Clotrimazole is available over the counter as a 1% solution in 10-mL bottles, and approximately 100 mL of solution is required to fill the nasal cavity and sinuses of a dog. Enilconazole is supplied as a concentrated commercial-grade solution (~27%), which is diluted to a 1, 2, or 5% solution prior to instillation in the nasal cavity. After the 1-hour infusion, the dog is placed in sternal recumbency to allow drainage of the drug. The oral cavity is rinsed clear of any medication because exposure of the drug to the mucosa can result in excessive soft tissue swelling and airway obstruction. This appears to be of more concern with enilconazole than clotrimazole.

Rhinoscopy should be performed in 1 month to evaluate response to therapy and confirm lack of fungal plaques because clinical signs and serology are not predictive of resolution of disease (Zonderland et al. 2002, Pomrantz and Johnson in press). Repeat treatment should be anticipated at the follow-up visit, and if fungal plaques are again present, a second recheck should be planned in 1 month.

Additional treatment methods have been reported including rhinotomy for debridement and instillation of clotrimazole cream into the frontal sinus to provide long-acting antifungal action. Clotrimazole cream is not retained within the region much longer than the standard solution used in treatment, although gel formulations are potentially promising for prolonged antifungal therapy (Mathews et al. 2009). If the integrity of the cribriform plate has been breached by infection, topical therapy is considered dangerous because of the possibility of toxic damage to the meninges from antifungal treatment. In these cases, oral therapy with voriconazole or posaconazole can be effective in controlling disease.

Prognosis

In the first several days posttreatment, it is common to see an exacerbation of signs, but these should resolve within 1–2 weeks of therapy. A 7–10-day course of a broad-spectrum antibiotic (such as amoxicillin–clavulanate) can be used if discharge persists. Dogs should have monthly rhinoscopic evaluation and treatment until resolution of disease, and most dogs will require two to four treatments. Unfortunately, some dogs are never cured and others can have recurrence or reinfection many months after apparent cure. Animals with severe destructive rhinitis often continue to have residual nasal discharge despite resolution of fungal infection because of abnormal nasal architecture and loss of normal defense mechanisms.

Feline Sinonasal and Sino-Orbital Aspergillosis

Pathophysiology

Aspergillus spp. (*fumigatus* and *niger*) and/or *Neosartorya* spp. are responsible for a devastating disease in cats that appears to begin within the nasal cavity, spread to the sinuses, and in some cases, invade the orbital region, causing extensive nasal signs as well as bony lysis and exophthalmos. Cats are systemically healthy, although the status of the nasal cavity is unclear. It has been hypothesized that viral destruction of turbinates or chronic rhinosinusitis may predispose some cats to development of fungal infection. Although much less common than the canine disease, more cats are being recognized with this syndrome.

History and signalment

Any age cat can be affected by aspergillosis and it appears that brachycephalic breeds are at increased risk. This is an interesting contrast to canine aspergillosis, which affects primarily dolicocephalic breeds. Presenting complaints are similar to those seen with idiopathic rhinitis or neoplasia, with unilateral or bilateral nasal discharge, epistaxis, and sneezing commonly reported. Signs may be present for weeks to years. Cats that develop extension of infection into the sinus or orbital region can develop facial distortion or a mass lesion.

Physical examination

Nasal depigmentation is not a feature of aspergillosis in cats, although ulceration of the hard palate or behind the last molar can be detected (Barrs et al. 2007). Cats with sinonasal disease can display obstruction of nasal airflow due to the presence of a nasal or nasopharyngeal granuloma, and cats with sino-orbital disease often have unilateral exophthalmos with protrusion of the third eyelid.

Diagnostic findings

Serology against fungal antigens by using counter-immunelectrophoresis, ELISA, or AGID has been positive in some cats diagnosed with aspergillosis; however, the sensitivity and specificity of these tests have not been examined. Fungal culture of a visually obtained sample from the plaque can be helpful in identifying the cause of disease; however, false negatives and false positives are common. In addition, culture alone cannot determine the infecting species as identification of *Neosartorya* requires PCR and sequencing.

A CT scan is helpful in determining the extent and severity of disease; however, imaging findings overlap with those seen with rhinitis and neoplasia. Variable degrees of turbinate lysis and collapse can be seen (Figure 4.12) along with soft tissue mass effects in the nasal cavity or nasopharynx. Importantly a CT scan can help define bone invasion and can determine whether both sides of the nasal cavity are involved. Rhinoscopic identification of granulomatous or plaque lesions (Figure 4.13) is helpful in solidifying the diagnosis because obtaining visualized biopsy samples allows confirmation of the presence of fungal organisms by cytology or histopathology.

Treatment

Optimal treatment in the cat is unknown, although success has been noted with topical clotrimazole and oral therapy with itraconazole, voriconazole, and posaconazole, with posaconazole showing the most promise. Debulking the fungal mass in cats with nasal or nasopharyngeal disease appears to be helpful. Severely affected animals or those that are poorly responsive to a single agent may respond to concurrent treatment with amophotericin B, liposomal amphotericin, or terbinafine. Cats with sino-orbital disease may require exenteration of the globe along with aggressive antifungal therapy. Optimal length of therapy has not been determined and several cats have relapsed when medications have been discontinued following resolution of clinical signs alone.

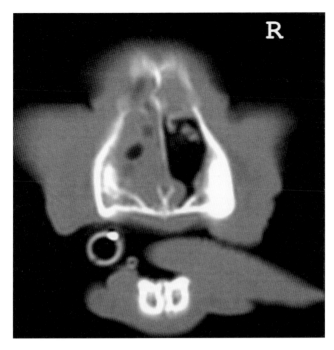

Figure 4.12. CT image of the rostral nasal cavity from a cat presented for a 2-month history of purulent nasal discharge. Cavitation and collapse of turbinates are noted on the right side of the nasal cavity. The left side is filled with soft tissue density and gas pocketing is noted. This appearance is consistent with lymphoma, severe chronic rhinitis, or granulomatous disease. Fungal hyphae consistent with *Aspergillus* spp. were found on histopathology.

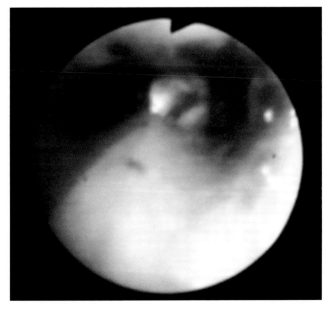

Figure 4.13. Retroflex view of the choanae in a 10-year-old FS Scottish Fold with a 4-year history of sneezing, epistaxis, and purulent nasal discharge. A fungal granuloma can be seen protruding into the nasopharynx. Histopathology revealed fungal hyphae.

Prognosis

Prognosis for sinonasal aspergillosis is difficult to determine given the few cases that have been reported in the literature, but some cats will respond to therapy over 3–10 months. Sino-orbital aspergillosis in the cat carries a grave prognosis for recovery, and many cats are euthanized following diagnosis.

Inflammatory Diseases

Nasopharyngeal Polyps

Pathophysiology

Nasal, nasopharyngeal, pharyngeal, or aural polyps are made up of fibrous inflammatory tissue that is suspected to originate from the Eustachian tube. A polyp can extend into the inner or middle ear, pharynx, or nasal cavity. They are found much more commonly in kittens than in puppies. Although an infectious etiology has been suspected, organisms have not been identified using culture or PCR (Veir et al. 2002).

History and signalment

Nasopharyngeal polyps are usually discovered in young animals, with the majority of affected patients under the age of 12 months; however, they may go undetected until the animal reaches adulthood. Nasal, pharyngeal, or nasopharyngeal polyps result in stertorous breathing, nasal discharge, dysphagia or dysphonia, gagging, and intermittent upper airway obstruction. Polyps in the ear canal lead to chronic aural discharge or head shaking. If otitis media is present, complaints may include a head tilt, ataxia, nystagmus, facial nerve paralysis, or Horner's syndrome.

Physical examination

Nasal or nasopharyngeal polyps lead to unilateral or bilateral loss of nasal airflow. A mass may be palpable in the nasopharynx above the soft palate. For animals with aural polyps, there may be evidence of otitis externa, a fluctuant polypoid mass in the ear canal, or a bulging tympanic membrane if middle ear disease is present.

Diagnostic findings

In cases that are suspicious for a polyp, lateral and dorsoventral radiographs of the pharyngeal region can suggest the presence of a polyp within the nasopharynx or of otitis media (Figure 4.14). CT scan should be considered prior to treatment since involvement of the tympanic bulla has been reported in 50–80% of cases and impacts the treatment most likely to be effective. If neurologic testing is performed, some cats can be found to be deaf at the time of diagnosis and owners should be aware that deafness will persist after surgery (Anders et al. 2008).

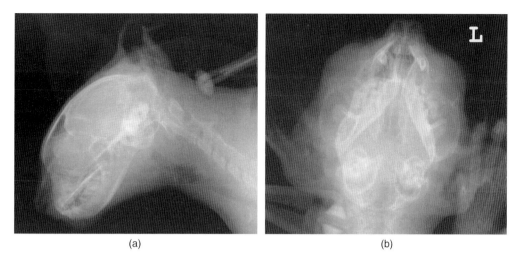

(a)   (b)

Figure 4.14. Radiographs from an 8-month old FS DSH presented for a 1-month history of congested breathing. Nasal airflow was absent bilaterally, and the lateral radiograph reveals a soft tissue density within the nasopharynx just ventral to the bulla (a). The dorsoventral radiograph shows asymmetry, with fluid filling of the right bulla and thickening of the bone consistent with right-sided otitis media (b).

Visual examination of the aural canal, pharynx, nasopharynx, or nasal cavity will often reveal the presence of a polyp; however, anesthesia is required. Evaluation of this area is most easily obtained with flexible endoscopy (Figure 4.15) although rostral retraction of the soft palate and use of a dental mirror can provide an appropriate view.

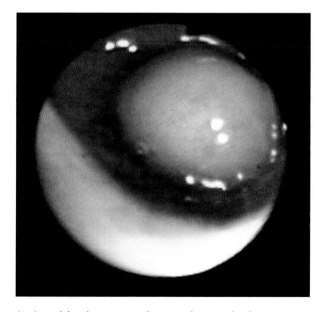

Figure 4.15. Endoscopic view of the choanae reveals a nasopharyngeal polyp.

Treatment

Traction and avulsion of the polyp from the stalk can be considered as an initial treatment option; however, in cats with bulla disease, a relatively high rate of recurrence may be found. With bulla involvement, treatment requires unilateral or bilateral bulla osteotomy with collection of samples for aerobic and anaerobic bacterial culture. Appropriate antibiotics are prescribed to treat middle ear disease. Removal of a large nasopharyngeal polyp may require a ventral midline approach through the palate.

Prognosis

Complications of surgery are not uncommon but are usually transient. These include Horner's syndrome (miosis, enophthalmos, and protrusion of the nictitans), which occurs in up to 80% of animals that undergo bulla osteotomy, and otitis interna with head tilt, ataxia, and nystagmus. Recurrence of the polyp is also possible and can occur in up to 50% of cats with bulla involvement that are treated by the retraction/avulsion technique (Veir et al. 2002).

Feline Chronic Rhinosinusitis

Pathophysiology

Chronic rhinosinusitis (CRS) is one of the most common chronic upper respiratory tract disorders seen in the feline population and is characterized by nasal discharge and sneezing associated with excessive mucus production. While various viral agents and bacteria are implicated as causes of acute upper respiratory tract disease of cats, the underlying pathogenesis in chronic feline rhinitis is less certain. The disease is likely multifactorial with viral (FHV-1) infection, secondary bacterial infection, and a poorly regulated or inappropriate local immune response contributing to the pathogenesis of disease.

History and signalment

Chronic rhinosinusitis affects all ages of cats, with clinical signs first apparent in cats anywhere from 6 months to 20 years of age. Stertor, mucopurulent or hemorrhagic nasal discharge, and sneezing are the most common historical complaints and clinical signs, and intermittent antibiotic responsiveness is common. Nasal discharge is often bilateral; however, some cases are remarkably unilateral. Ocular and systemic signs are usually absent, in comparison to the disease in kittens with acute upper respiratory tract infection.

Physical examination

Nasal discharge may not be apparent on physical examination because cats are fastidious groomers; however, sneezing may be observed. Cats with CRS generally have preservation of nasal airflow, in comparison to cats with neoplasia or fungal infection in which airflow is obstructed. Soft palate and ocular compression are normal and it is uncommon to detect regional lymphadenopathy, although this can be seen rarely. The remainder of the physical examination is usually unremarkable, and cats are systemically well.

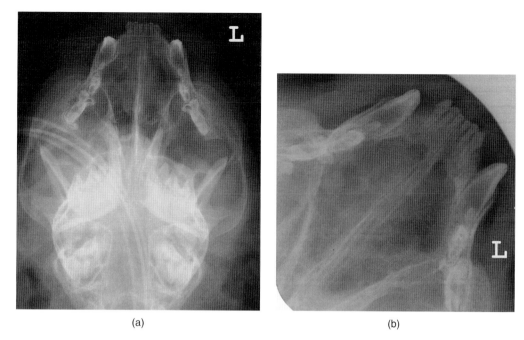

(a)   (b)

Figure 4.16. Open mouth views of the nasal cavity of a cat taken under general anesthesia obtained with conventional skull radiography (a) and dental radiography (b). Skull radiographs are obtained in dorsal recumbency with the jaw retracted, while the dental radiograph is obtained in sternal recumbency with the radiographic film placed in the mouth. Mild asymmetry is seen between the two sides of the nasal cavity with an increase in soft tissue or fluid density on the right.

Diagnostic findings

The diagnosis of chronic rhinosinusitis is one of exclusion, and owners should be made aware of this prior to initiating expensive and somewhat invasive diagnostic testing. The approach involves an assessment of the extent of systemic illness with a minimum database. Cytology of nasal discharge and/or a cryptococcal antigen test can be performed to rule out cryptococcosis in appropriate situations. In cats with hemorrhagic nasal discharge, blood pressure evaluation and a coagulation panel should be performed.

Anesthesia is required for additional diagnostics. Skull radiographs show variable degrees of turbinate lysis and increased fluid density within the nasal cavity. The open mouth dorsoventral view or dental radiographs provide the best visualization of the nasal cavity (Figure 4.16) and a CT scan provides better visualization of intranasal structures (Figure 4.17). Sinuses or the middle ear is sometimes involved in the disease process or may be fluid filled (Figure 4.18). The severity of radiographic or tomographic changes overlap with those typically found in nasal neoplasia, making biopsy differentiation crucial.

Rhinoscopy with biopsy is performed after imaging has been completed to avoid causing hemorrhage that would alter the radiologic appearance of the nasal cavity. First, nasopharyngoscopy is accomplished by retroflex of a flexible endoscope above the soft palate to rule out nasopharyngeal stenosis or a mass lesion. Rostral rhinoscopy of the nasal cavity typically reveals hyperemic mucosa, variable amounts of mucoid to purulent discharge, and

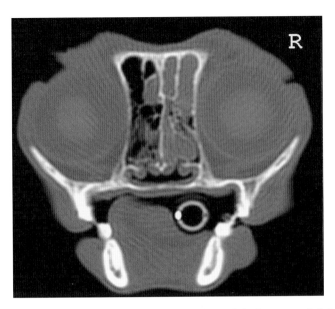

Figure 4.17. CT image of the nasal cavity in a cat with right-sided nasal discharge reveals fluid accumulation and some gas pocketing.

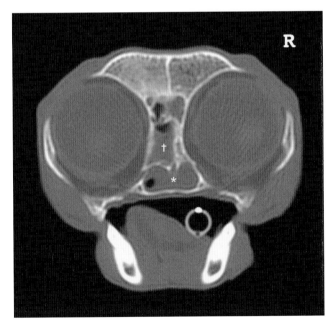

Figure 4.18. CT image through the frontal sinus and nasopharyngeal region of a 2-year-old FS DSH with lifelong nasal congestion. Note the absence of air in the frontal sinuses and replacement by fibrous or bony tissue. The sphenopalatine sinuses are distorted (†) and filled with soft tissue density as is the nasopharynx (*).

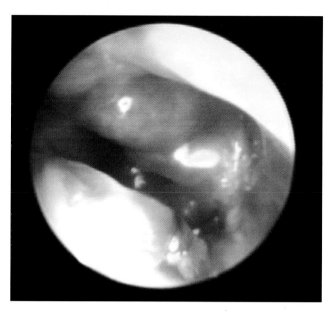

Figure 4.19. Rhinoscopic image in a cat with CRS reveals moderate mucosal hyperemia, blunting of turbinates, and destructive rhinitis (visible as increased space within the nasal cavity). Thick mucoid discharge is evident ventrally.

irregular turbinate structures (Figure 4.19), although some affected cats will have minimal visual changes. Rhinoscopic appearance does not predict the presence or absence of substantial inflammation, and bilateral nasal biopsy (using 2- or 3-mm cup biopsy forceps) is recommended to assess the type and severity of inflammation. Histologic evidence of nasal inflammation is virtually always present in cats with CRS, with the majority of severe cases demonstrating neutrophilic inflammation indicative of an acute component to the disease. Lymphoplasmacytic inflammation indicates chronicity while eosinophilic infiltrates may indicate FHV-1-related disease (Hargis et al. 1999).

Obtaining a deep flush or brush sample from the caudal nasal cavity for bacterial culture (aerobic, anaerobic, and *Mycoplasma*) can be helpful in guiding antibiotic therapy as cats with chronic rhinitis have potential pathogens isolated from nasal samples more commonly than do normal cats (Johnson et al. 2005). Extensive nasal flushing after completion of sample collection (see Chapter 2) can improve response to therapy by removing excessive mucus and inflammatory debris from the nasal cavity. After rhinoscopy, dental probing is performed to identify oronasal fistulae or large periodontal pockets that could be responsible for dental-related nasal disease.

Treatment

Antibiotics
Chronic antibiotic therapy is usually employed to control secondary bacterial rhinitis. Choice of antibiotics for the individual cat can be based on culture of a deep nasal flush or brush sample, or may be made with an understanding of potential pathogens that have been isolated previously from cats with rhinitis. Those organisms include aerobes (*Pasteurella multocida, E. coli, Corynebacterium ulcerans, Bordetella bronchiseptica, Streptococcus*

viridans, Pseudomonas aeruginosa, Actinomyces slackii), anaerobes (*Peptostreptococcus anaerobius, Bacteroides fragilis, B. ureolyticus, Prevotella, Fusobacterium nucleatum*), and *Mycoplasma felis* (Johnson et al. 2005). Doxycycline (approximately 50 mg/cat PO divided every 12 hours or given once daily) is an appropriate antibiotic to use because it has efficacy against these bacteria. In addition, doxycycline may help control clinical signs through anti-inflammatory or immunomodulatory effects. Doxycycline is well tolerated by most cats even when administered for a long term, and it is inexpensive. The primary caution with use of this drug is the potential for development of an esophageal stricture if the pill lodges in the esophagus. Instruction labels should always contain the recommendation to follow administration of the pill with a small volume (5–6 mL) of water.

Other commonly used antibiotics include azithromycin, cephalexin, and amoxicillin–clavulanic acid. Azithromycin is an appealing option for long-term therapy. It is available as a powder for oral suspension and can be given once daily (5 mg/kg for 3–5 days followed by twice weekly administration) because it accumulates in tissue. This antibiotic is also reported to have anti-inflammatory and tissue repair effects. Penicillin-like drugs are helpful in controlling signs in many cats although they lack efficacy against *Mycoplasma* species. They are also frequently associated with gastrointestinal side effects. Enrofloxacin (Baytril [Bayer], 2.5 mg/kg PO every 24 hours) is generally reserved for infections that are susceptible to this antibiotic, and high doses should be avoided since they have been associated with retinopathy. Clindamycin can be efficacious in cases with extensive bony involvement because of its ability to penetrate bone. Antibiotic treatment is usually continued for at least 3–6 weeks on the basis of the assumption that deep-seated infection is present. Intermittent or suppressive long-term antibiotic therapy may be required.

Anti-inflammatory agents

Nonspecific nasal inflammation can be treated with piroxicam at 0.3 mg/kg PO daily or every other day. This drug is commercially available as a 10-mg tablet, and drug compounding is required. This nonsteroidal anti-inflammatory agent causes subclinical gastric erosion, and caution is warranted in its use in older animals or in cats with renal insufficiency. In some instances, a gastrointestinal protectant (famotidine) or prostaglandin analog (misoprostol) might be administered concurrently; however, it can be difficult giving multiple oral medications to a cat chronically. Meloxicam is a tempting alternative to piroxicam because it is easier to dose and administer, although subjectively, cats do not appear to respond as well to that drug.

Glucocorticoids are sometimes advocated for treatment of cats with CRS, and in some animals with excessive mucus in the nasal cavity, administration of oral steroids may reduce mucus accumulation and promote appetite. Caution is warranted if eosinophilic nasal inflammation is detected or if FHV-1-related ocular disease is present because steroids can result in exacerbation of disease. Inhaled or topical steroids are also sometimes advocated, although mucus must be cleared from the nasal cavity prior to use to allow absorption by the mucosal surface. Metered-dose inhaler preparations containing steroids require administration with a spacer chamber and facemask. Liquid steroid medications are available in drop formulations or as nasal sprays and are variably tolerated.

Antiviral therapy

The role of FHV-1 in induction or promotion of clinical signs in cats with CRS has not been clearly established, and specific antiviral therapy is not recommended in cats with chronic disease. Trial therapy with lysine can be considered in a cat with CRS as this amino acid reduces viral replication by competing with arginine for use by FHV-1 in protein synthesis. Lysine would be particularly indicated when intranuclear inclusions or an eosinophilic inflammatory infiltrate is reported on histology. The recommended dose of lysine is 500 mg/cat PO BID, and this dose does not result in a drop in serum arginine levels in the cat. Lysine can be purchased at most health food stores as a pill or a capsule containing granules, and veterinary paste formulations are also available. Current research has shown that famcyclovir is efficacious against FHV-1-related ocular disease and there may be a role for this drug in treatment of cats with CRS if an etiologic role for viral infection is confirmed.

Additional therapy

Rigorous flushing of the nasal cavity when the animal is anesthetized for diagnostic testing improves the clinical response of cats with CRS (see Chapter 2). Cats can also benefit from intermittent airway humidification via steam inhalation or nebulization. Oral administration of N-acetylcysteine (150–250 mg/cat PO BID) can help some cats by reducing the viscosity of secretions and encouraging evacuation of the nasal cavity.

Prognosis

Most cats with chronic rhinosinusitis have severe abnormalities in nasal and sinus structure and function, and it is unlikely that disease can be abolished in these cats. Owners should be aware that clinical signs of disease can be controlled to a variable extent but animals are rarely cured. Some cats have recurrent episodes of sneezing and nasal discharge despite long-term therapy, and a reasonable goal of therapy is to limit the severity and frequency of disease exacerbations.

Canine Lymphoplasmacytic Rhinitis

Pathophysiology

Histologic evidence of lymphoplasmacytic nasal inflammation can be found in conjunction with primary neoplastic, fungal, or foreign body rhinitis. Idiopathic lymphoplasmacytic rhinitis (LPR) is a condition that lacks a primary source of the inflammatory infiltrate. This condition has been referred to as immune-mediated or allergic rhinitis because initial reports suggested that steroid therapy was curative; however, more recent studies suggest that steroids are not universally effective. Many dogs display a transient response to antibiotic therapy; however, clinical signs return when the drugs are withdrawn or sometimes recur in the face of treatment. Increased fungal DNA has been found in nasal tissue of dogs with LPR (Windsor et al. 2006), and a partial Th2 cytokine response has been described locally (Peeters et al. 2007). These results might be suggestive of a fungal hypersensitivity but further work is required to establish the etiology.

History and signalment

Idiopathic LPR generally affects young to middle-aged, large-breed mesaticephalic dogs. Males and females are equally affected. Nasal discharge (unilateral or bilateral) is the most common clinical complaint in dogs with LPR. Discharge is typically mucoid or mucopurulent in most dogs but can be serous, and hemorrhagic or blood-tinged discharge is not uncommon. Interestingly, some dogs may present with true epistaxis rather than nasal discharge. Other possible clinical signs include sneezing, coughing, reverse sneezing, stertorous breathing, ocular discharge, and pawing/rubbing at the muzzle.

Physical examination

Nasal airflow is generally preserved in dogs with LPR and the remainder of the physical examination is often unremarkable. Some dogs with LPR may have regional lymphadenopathy due to reactive lymphoid hyperplasia. Careful thoracic auscultation is recommended because some dogs with signs suggestive of LPR may have concurrent lower airway disease with regurgitation of secretions into the nasopharynx.

Diagnostic findings

Laboratory testing is unremarkable in affected dogs, and testing for *Bartonella* organisms has not revealed a role for these organisms in idiopathic nasal disease (Hawkins et al. 2008). Nasal radiography has low sensitivity for differentiating inflammatory rhinitis from neoplasia or mycotic rhinitis because soft tissue opacification, turbinate destruction, and frontal sinus disease can be seen with all three conditions. A CT scan provides improved definition of the extent and severity of abnormalities in the nasal cavity, although LPR can cause CT lesions that mimic those found with these other conditions (Figure 4.20). Turbinate destruction is found commonly, although it is generally mild or moderate in most cases. Fluid accumulation, soft tissue opacification, gas pocketing, and frontal sinus involvement are also common CT findings, and abnormalities can be unilateral or bilateral.

Rhinoscopy typically reveals hyperemic, friable, inflamed epithelium and mucus accumulation (Figure 4.21). Mild turbinate destruction is sometimes seen. Biopsy samples reveal lymphoplasmacytic infiltrates of varying severity reflecting the chronicity of disease, mucosal edema, and bony remodeling of turbinates. Culture of a nasal swab or flush is rarely of use, but when submitted, samples generally display only minimal growth of bacterial flora.

Treatment

Treatment options for idiopathic LPR are limited because the etiology of the disorder remains unclear. Modulatory antimicrobial therapy with long-term doxycycline or azithromycin, or anti-inflammatory treatment with piroxicam (0.3 mg/kg PO daily) can be helpful in some dogs, although a guarded prognosis for cure must be given. Some response has been anecdotally reported for alternate therapies (oral itraconazole and inhaled steroids), although specific information is lacking. Airway humidification or nebulization or oral administration of N-acetylcysteine can help liquefy nasal secretions and may be beneficial in some cases.

Prognosis

The etiology of LPR remains obscure, and therefore, the efficacy of specific drug therapy cannot be determined. Although not life threatening, owner tolerance of the disorder can be limited.

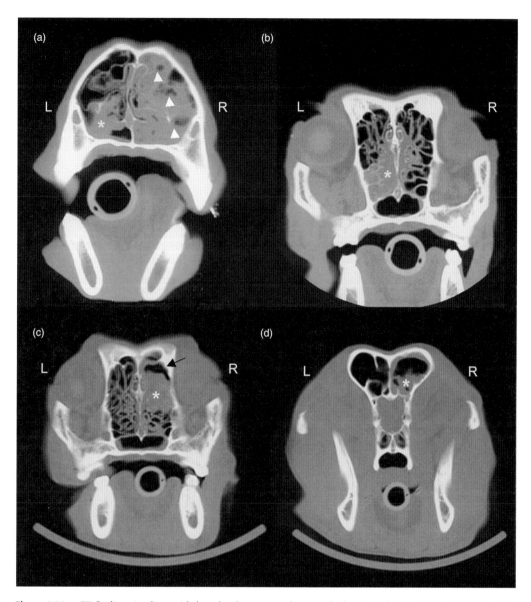

Figure 4.20. CT findings in dogs with lymphoplasmacytic rhinitis. Fluid accumulation in the right side of the nasal cavity is evident, along with gas pocketing of the fluid (white arrowheads). A small amount of fluid (*) in the ventral aspect of the left nasal cavity is also seen (a). Fluid is seen around the rostral aspect of the cribriform (*) without evidence of destruction (b). Fluid forms a relatively well-defined mass lesion in the right nasal cavity (*), and there is mild turbinate loss dorsal to the region of fluid accumulation (black arrow) (c). Fluid accumulation in the right frontal sinus (*) and thickening of the mucosa associated with the dorsum of the frontal sinus is evident (d). (Reprinted with permission from the *Journal of the American Medical Association* (Windsor 2004.)

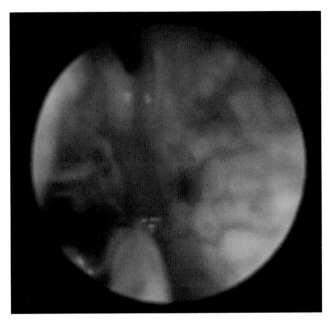

Figure 4.21. Rhinoscopic image from a dog with idiopathic LPR reveals mucosal hyperemia, mucus accumulation, and irregular turbinate structures.

Nasal Neoplasia

Pathophysiology

Nasal tumors represent a small percentage of neoplasms in cats and dogs; however, the majority of cases exhibit malignant behavior through local invasion and extension. Tumor types encountered include lymphosarcoma, adenocarcinoma, squamous cell carcinoma, undifferentiated carcinoma or sarcoma, fibrosarcoma, chondrosarcoma, and osteosarcoma. Lymphosarcoma appears to be the most common nasal neoplasm in the cat. The biologic behavior of most nasal tumors is characterized by local extension; however, metastasis to regional lymph nodes is relatively common and impacts treatment options. Metastasis to the lung is rare. Nasal lymphoma in the cat may be associated with systemic disease at the time of diagnosis or some cats may develop systemic lymphoma during or after treatment of nasal disease (Haney et al. 2009).

History and signalment

Nasal neoplasia is primarily a disease of older dogs and cats; however, young to middle-aged animals (2–5 years) can also be affected. Clinical complaints are similar to those seen with other nasal disorders and include sneezing, epistaxis, stertorous respirations, or nasal discharge. Discharge is usually unilateral initially but may become bilateral when the vomer bone is breached. Some animals are presented because of difficulty breathing through the nose or open mouth breathing. Neurologic abnormalities such as seizures, behavioral

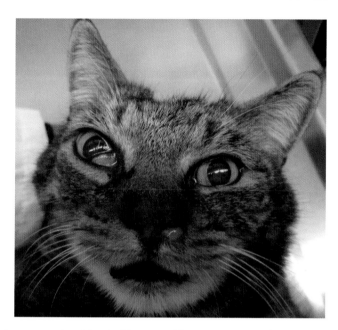

Figure 4.22. Facial asymmetry is evident in this 9-year-old MC DSH presented for evaluation of nasal discharge. The right eye is displaced laterally and dorsally by a mass effect. Tear staining is evident OD and the nictitating membrane is elevated. Necropsy revealed lymphoma filling the right nasal cavity, nasopharynx, and retrobulbar space with extension into the olfactory lobe and cerebrum.

changes, or cerebral dysfunction can be seen alone or in conjunction with respiratory signs. The presence of these signs is highly suggestive of tumor invasion into the central nervous system and warrants a guarded prognosis.

Physical examination

Nasal discharge (unilateral or bilateral) with loss of nasal airflow is a common finding. Facial deformity, unilateral epiphora, or a mass protruding from the nostrils seem to occur more commonly in cats than in dogs (Figure 4.22). Nasal tumors can result in differential ocular retropulsion when the tumor grows up the optic tract. When neoplasms extend caudally, they can sometimes be felt above the soft palate in the nasopharyngeal region. Regional lymphadenopathy is an important clinical finding because this is a common site for metastasis. It is important to remember, however, that metastasis can be present in the absence of palpable lymph node enlargement.

Diagnostic findings

Laboratory tests are usually unremarkable. Fine-needle aspiration of the lymph node ipsilateral to the discharge is recommended because cytology may reveal neoplastic cells and provide a diagnosis prior to more expensive or invasive diagnostics.

Skull radiographs reveal unilateral or bilateral increased soft tissue density in the nasal cavity, destruction of turbinate structures, or vomer lysis. The frontal sinus may be filled

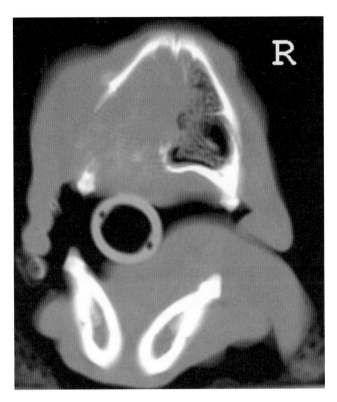

Figure 4.23. CT image from a 9-year-old FS Doberman with a 2-month history of left-sided epistaxis. An expansile soft tissue mass with regions of mineralization fills the rostral left nasal cavity. There is erosion of the maxilla and hard palate on the left side and erosion through the septum into the right nasal cavity. Histopathology confirmed nasal osteosarcoma.

with soft tissue or fluid density or a fluid line may be visible. This can indicate either tumor in the sinus or fluid accumulation due to obstruction. A CT scan is more useful than radiography for determining tumor boundaries, assessing the integrity of the cribriform plate to detect central nervous system involvement, and planning radiation therapy (Figure 4.23). Rhinoscopy typically reveals a mass lesion protruding between the turbinates (Figure 4.24), although in some cases, swollen or deformed turbinates may be seen. Obtaining a biopsy sample while visualizing the abnormal region rhinoscopically is important for confirming the diagnosis with histopathology.

Treatment

The most commonly employed treatment of nasal tumors is radiation therapy because surgery does not resolve signs or result in improved survival. Chemotherapeutic protocols are under investigation. Palliation of clinical signs can be achieved by use of piroxicam (0.3 mg/kg/day). Addition of cyclophosphamide (10 mg/m^2 daily to every other day) for metronomic chemotherapy might improve clinical response. Nasal lymphosarcoma in the cat is treated with standard chemotherapeutic protocols for lymphoma, radiation therapy, or a combination of the two treatment modalities.

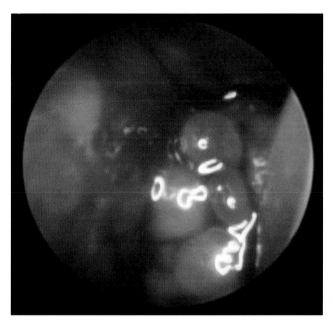

Figure 4.24. Rhinoscopic image from a dog with nasal neoplasia reveals a soft tissue mass protruding between turbinates in the nasal cavity.

Prognosis

The goal of radiation therapy is to control or limit clinical signs. In dogs, median survival times of 9–23 months have been reported for various tumors by using different protocols and types of radiation. Side effects of radiation therapy are predictable and expected because the radiation dose required to kill tumor cells will kill normal cells that undergo rapid cell division, such as epithelial cells. Early side effects include mucositis, conjunctivitis, and moist desquamation of skin. Ocular lubricants can be used, but specific treatment of the skin is not recommended. If mucositis causes anorexia, cold tea mouth rinses may make the animal more comfortable. In severe cases, an esophageal tube should be considered to provide nutrition. Late effects of radiation therapy are generally irreversible and include bone necrosis, cataracts, and keratoconjunctivitis sicca.

Cats with nasal or nasopharyngeal lymphoma may experience up to 2.5 years of progression-free disease and prolonged survival when treated with radiation and/or chemotherapy, although systemic disease may develop despite local control (Sfiligoi et al. 2007, Haney et al. 2009). It appears that inclusion of local radiation treatment may improve median survival time due to better control of tumor growth, with higher doses resulting in longer duration of local disease control (Haney et al. 2009).

References

Anders BB, Hoelzler MG, Scavelli TD, et al. Analysis of auditory and neurologic effects associated with ventral bulla osteotomy for removal of inflammatory polyps or nasopharyngeal masses in cats. J Am Vet Med Assoc. 2008; 233: 580–585.

Barrs VR, Martin P, Beatty JA, et al. Feline sino-orbital aspergillosis, an emerging clinical syndrome. J Vet Int Med. 2007, 21: 579 (abstract).

Berent AC, Weisse C, Todd K, et al. Use of a balloon-expandable metallic stent for treatment of nasopharyngeal stenosis in dogs and cats: six cases (2005–2007). J Am Vet Med Assoc. 2008; 233: 1432–1440.

De Lorenzi D, Bonfanti U, Masserdotti C, et al. Diagnosis of canine nasal aspergillosis by cytological examination: a comparison of four different collection techniques. J Small Anim Pract. 2006; 47: 316–319.

Ginn JA, Kumar MS, McKiernan BC, Powers BE. Nasopharyngeal turbinates in brachycephalic dogs and cats. J Am Anim Hosp Assoc. 2008; 44: 243–249.

Haney SM, Beaver L, Turrel J, et al. Survival analysis of 97 cats with nasal lymphoma: a multi-institutional retrospective study (1986–2006). J Vet Int Med. 2009; 23: 287–294.

Hargis AM, Ginn PE, Mansell JEKL, Garber RL. Ulcerative facial and nasal dermatitis and stomatitis associated with feline herpesvirus 1. Vet Dermatol. 1999; 10: 267–274.

Harvey CE, Fink EA. Tracheal diameter: analysis in brachycephalic and non-brachycephalic dogs. J Am Anim Hosp Assoc. 1982; 18: 570–576.

Hawkins EC, Johnson LR, Guptill L, et al. Failure to identify an association between serologic or molecular evidence of *Bartonella* spp. infection and idiopathic rhinitis in dogs. J Am Vet Med Assoc. 2008; 233: 597–599.

Hurley KE, Pesavento PA, Pedersen NC, Poland AM, Wilson E, Foley JE. An outbreak of virulent systemic feline calicivirus disease. J Am Vet Med Assoc. 2004; 224: 241–249.

Johnson LR, Drazenovich TL, Herrera MA, Wisner ER. Results of rhinoscopy alone or in conjunction with sinuscopy in dogs with aspergillosis: 46 cases (2001–2004). J Am Vet Med Assoc. 2006; 228: 738–742.

Johnson LR, Foley JE, De Cock HEV, et al. Assessment of infectious organisms associated with chronic rhinosinusitis in cats. J Am Vet Med Assoc. 2005; 227: 579–585.

Maggs DJ, Lappin MR, Reif JS, et al. Evaluation of serologic and viral detection methods for diagnosing feline herpesvirus-1 infection in cats with acute respiratory tract or chronic ocular disease. J Am Vet Med Assoc. 1999; 214: 502–507.

Maggs DJ, Sykes JE, Clarke HE, Yoo SH, Kass PH, Lappin MR, Rogers QR, Waldron MK, Fascetti AJ. Effects of dietary lysine supplementation in cats with enzootic upper respiratory disease. J Feline Med Surg. 2007; 9: 97–108.

Malik R, Craig AJ, Wigney DI, et al. Combination chemotherapy of canine and feline cryptococcosis using subcutaneously administered amphotericin B. Aust Vet J. 1996; 73: 124–128.

Malik R, Wigney DI, Muir DB, et al. Cryptococcosis in cats: clinical and mycological assessment of 29 cases and evaluation of treatment using orally administered fluconazole. J Med Vet Mycol. 1992; 30: 133–144.

Mathews KG, Linder KE, Davidson GS, et al. Assessment of clotrimazole gels for in vitro stability and in vivo retention in the frontal sinus of dogs. Am J Vet Res. 2009; 70: 640–647.

Medleau L, Jacobs GJ, Marks MA. Itraconazole for treatment of cryptococcosis in cats. J Vet Int Med. 1995; 9: 39–42.

O'Brien CR, Krockenberger MB, Martin P, et al. Long-term outcome of therapy for 59 cats and 11 dogs with cryptococcosis. Aust Vet J. 2006; 84: 384–392.

Pedersen NC, Sato R, Foley JE, Poland AM. Common virus infections in cats, before and after being placed in shelters, with emphasis on feline enteric coronavirus. J Feline Med Surg. 2004; 6 (2): 83–88.

Peeters D, Peters IR, Clercx C, Day MJ. Quantification of mRNA encoding cytokines and chemokines in nasal biopsies from dogs with sino-nasal aspergillosis. Vet Microbiol. 2006; 31; 114: 318–326.

Peeters D, Peters IR, Helps CR, et al. Distinct tissue cytokine and chemokine mRNA expression in canine sino-nasal aspergillosis and idiopathic lymphoplasmacytic rhinitis. Vet Immunol Immunopathol. 2007; 117 (1–2): 95–105.

Pomrantz JS, Johnson LR. Rhinoscopic and serologic assessment of disease in dogs with nasal aspergillosis. J Am Vet Med Assoc. in press.

Pomrantz JS, Johnson LR, Nelson RW, Wisner ER. Utility of Aspergillus serology and tissue fungal culture in canine nasal disease. J Am Vet Med Assoc. 2007; 230: 1319–1323.

Poncet CM, Dupre GP, Freiche VG, et al. Prevalence of gastrointestinal tract lesions in 73 brachycephalic dogs with upper respiratory syndrome. J Small Anim Pract. 2005; 46: 273–279.

Poncet CM, Dupre GM, Freiche VG, et al. Long-term results of upper respiratory syndrome surgery and gastrointestinal tract medical treatment in 51 brachycephalic dogs. J Small Anim Pract. 2006; 47: 137–142.

Sfiligoi G, Théon AP, Kent MS. Response of nineteen cats with nasal lymphoma to radiation therapy and chemotherapy. Vet Radiol Ultrasound. 2007; 48: 388–393.

Smith AW, Iversen PL, O'Hanley PD, et al. Virus-specific antiviral treatment for controlling severe and fatal outbreaks of feline calicivirus infection. Am J Vet Res. 2008; 69: 23–32.

Suter PF. A Text Atlas of Thoracic Diseases of the Dog and Cat. Wettswil, Switzerland. 1984, pp. 238–140.

Veir J, MR Lappin, JE Foley, DM Getzy. Feline inflammatory polyps: Historical, clinical, and PCR findings for feline calici virus and feline herpes virus-1 in 28 cases. J Feline Med Surg. 2002; 4: 195–199.

Windsor RC, Johnson LR, Herrgesell EJ, De Cock HEV. Lymphoplasmacytic rhinitis in 37 dogs: 1997–2002. J Am Vet Med Assoc. 2004; 224: 1952–1957.

Windsor RC, Johnson LR, JE Sykes, et al. Molecular detection of microbes in nasal tissue of dogs with idiopathic lymphoplasmacytic rhinitis. J Vet Int Med. 2006; 20: 250–256.

Zonderland JL, Stork CK, Saunders JH, et al. Intranasal infusion of enilconazole for treatment of sinonasal aspergillosis in dogs. J Am Vet Med Assoc. 2002; 221: 1421–1425.

Diseases of Airways

Structural Disorders

Laryngeal Paralysis

Pathophysiology

In normal animals, the dorsal cricoarytenoideus muscles contract to abduct the corniculate processes of the arytenoids during inspiration. This muscle is innervated by the recurrent laryngeal nerve, a branch of the vagus that originates near the thoracic inlet and loops around the subclavian artery on the right or the aorta on the left and returns craniad to the larynx. Laryngeal paralysis is recognized as a congenital disorder or as an acquired form in older, large-breed dogs. In the congenital disease in some breeds and in the acquired idiopathic form, laryngeal paralysis can be accompanied by a more generalized polyneuropathy that results in peripheral limb weakness. Electromyographic studies and nerve conduction velocities in peripheral limb musculature of dogs with acquired laryngeal paralysis are suggestive of axonal disease; however, it is unclear whether the neuromuscular supply to the larynx is affected by a similar disease process (Jeffrey et al. 2006). Laryngeal paralysis can also result from trauma via surgery (thyroidectomy or tracheal ring placement), bite wounds, or crush injuries. A mediastinal mass compressing the recurrent laryngeal nerve can also lead to laryngeal paralysis.

In animals with laryngeal paralysis, active contracture to open the glottis is depressed or lost, and this can be unilateral or bilateral. Inspiration against a narrowed glottis results in a pressure drop across the larynx, and turbulent velocity of airflow results in irritation of the mucosa. This leads to mucosal edema and further obstruction of airflow. The larynx serves as an important protective mechanism against pulmonary inhalation of damaging substances. It appears that some dogs with laryngeal dysfunction experience sensory as well as motor loss and this may result in silent aspiration of oropharyngeal or gastroesophageal contents. It is common for dogs with laryngeal paralysis to accumulate secretions around the glottis, resulting in gagging or retching.

Cats are also affected by congenital or acquired laryngeal paralysis but it is less commonly recognized clinically because they are less physically active and regulate activity to avoid respiratory distress associated with inspiratory obstruction.

History and signalment

Laryngeal paralysis results in inspiratory difficulty, dysphonia, excessive or loud panting, gagging, and retching. Exercise intolerance may be the first abnormality noted, and can be mistaken as a sign of aging in the Retriever breeds. Signs are worsened by heat, stress, excitement, or exercise, and severely affected animals may suffer syncope or cyanosis. Careful questioning of the owner is recommended to uncover concurrent esophageal or gastrointestinal dysfunction because the combination of regurgitation or vomiting with laryngeal disease or laryngeal surgery enhances the risk for aspiration pneumonia.

Congenital laryngeal paralysis has been reported in several breeds of dogs and can be associated with additional neurologic deficits in some breeds (Table 5.1). Purebred animals with congenital disease are young when signs are first recognized, although the disease in Shepherds and Leonbergers has a later onset. The acquired form results in clinical signs late in life (10–14 years of age), and traumatic or iatrogenic injury to the larynx during surgery can result in development of signs at any age.

Physical examination

In some animals, upper airway auscultation is difficult because of continual panting. Inspiratory stridor audible over the larynx is the classic finding on physical examination; however, this may be a subtle finding in some dogs. Gently exercising the patient to increase respiratory effort may elicit stridorous sounds; however, caution is warranted to avoid overheating. Some large-breed dogs, particularly those that are obese, can develop life-threatening hyperthermia caused by excessive work of breathing.

Dogs with generalized neuromuscular disease can also display limb weakness exhibited by decreased conscious proprioception or patellar reflexes, and less commonly, a depressed gag or tongue reflex can be detected (Jeffrey et al. 2006). A full neurologic assessment is important in dogs with idiopathic laryngeal paralysis because these dogs may suffer continued weakness or exercise intolerance after surgical treatment of the larynx.

Diagnostic findings

There are no specific laboratory findings associated with laryngeal paralysis. A complete blood count (CBC) should be screened for neutrophilic leukocytosis suggestive of aspiration pneumonia, and a chemistry panel and urinalysis are performed to exclude systemic disease. Several studies have ruled out an association of thyroid dysfunction with laryngeal paralysis and testing is not advocated unless concurrent signs suggest hypothyroidism. If an arterial blood gas is performed, mild hypoxemia might be detected but the more obvious finding anticipated is hypercapnea associated with alveolar hypoventilation (see Chapter 2). In a dog with normal lung function, the alveolar-to-arterial ratio should be normal.

Table 5.1. Congenital forms of laryngeal paralysis

Breed	Age of Onset	Sex	Mode of Inheritance	Additional Findings	Reference
Dalmatian	2–6 months	Male = female	Autosomal recessive	Megaesophagus Polyneuropathy	Braund et al. (1994)
Rottweiler	9–13 weeks	Male > female	Unknown	Polyneuropathy Cataracts	Mahoney et al. (1998)
Great Pyrenees	2–6 months		Autosomal recessive (postulated)	Megaesophagus Polyneuropathy	Gabriel et al. (2006)
Bouvier des Flandres	4–6 months	Male > female	Autosomal dominant	Neuronal degeneration in the recurrent laryngeal nerve	Venker van-Haagen et al. (1978)
Siberian Husky and mix	4–6 months		Unknown		O'Brien et al. (1986)
White German Shepherd	9–24 months		Possibly linked to white haircoat		Ridyard et al. (2000)
Leonberger	1–3 years	Male	X-linked with partial penetration	Polyneuropathy	Shelton et al. (2003)

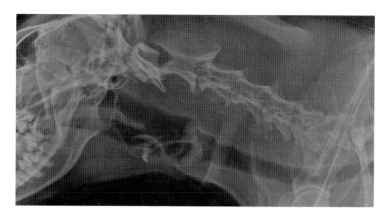

Figure 5.1.   This right lateral cervical radiograph of a 9-year-old MC Labrador Retriever with stridor reveals caudal retraction of the larynx and hyoid apparatus consistent with an upper airway obstruction.

Differential diagnosis for laryngeal paralysis includes laryngeal neoplasia, granuloma, foreign body, or inflammatory laryngitis. Cervical radiographs can be helpful in ruling out a laryngeal mass, and indirect evidence of upper airway obstruction can be seen as caudal retraction of the larynx (Figure 5.1). Experienced examiners can document deficient laryngeal motion during ultrasound examination. Chest radiographs are recommended to assess the esophagus and to document evidence of aspiration pneumonia. If vomiting or regurgitation is in the history, videofluoroscopic assessment of esophageal function should be considered because defective function could impact the decision for anesthesia and surgery.

Diagnosis of laryngeal paralysis requires visualization of laryngeal motion under a light plane of anesthesia. The animal is placed in sternal recumbency, and a barbiturate anesthetic agent or propofol is administered to the dose that allows the mouth to be opened safely while preserving respiratory maneuvers. An assistant identifies inspiratory effort while the examiner watches for abduction of the arytenoids. If appropriate laryngeal function is not visualized initially, doxapram hydrochloride (0.5–2.2 mg/kg) can be administered intravenously as a bolus to stimulate respiration. Additional anesthesia is usually required at this point because doxapram can be stimulatory. It is important to time laryngeal motion with inspiratory effort because paradoxical laryngeal motion, where the larynx is pulled inwards by inspiratory effort and then passively opens on expiration, can be mistaken for normal motion. In addition to lack of motion, signs of laryngeal inflammation are often present in animals with laryngeal paralysis, such as hyperemia and accumulation of secretions around the larynx (Figure 5.2).

Dogs with laryngeal disease are at risk for aspiration pneumonia, which is augmented by respiratory depression associated with anesthesia. Therefore, it is prudent to plan for surgical intervention at the time of diagnostic laryngoscopy, if potential complications have been discussed with the client.

Treatment

Dogs and cats with unilateral laryngeal paralysis can usually tolerate the degree of dysfunction that results from partial airway obstruction and are not candidates for surgery. Weight loss and restricted activity during hot or humid weather should be recommended.

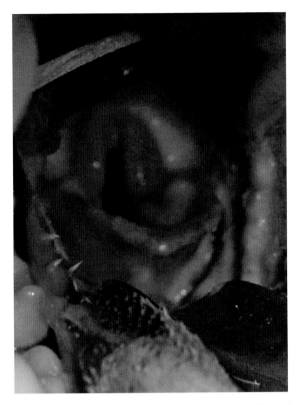

Figure 5.2.   This endoscopic image of an 11-year-old MC Labrador Retriever shows dramatic hyperemia of the larynx and accumulation of mucoid secretions lateral to the larynx and ventral to the epiglottis.

For animals with bilateral laryngeal paralysis, the decision to go to surgery is based on the quality of life of the dog, the severity of clinical signs, and the time of the year. It can be prudent to perform surgery when approaching the summer to allow sufficient recovery before hot weather develops because warmer weather causes dogs to breathe harder despite less physical exertion. This leads to worsened inflammation and edema, augmenting airway obstruction. Unilateral arytenoid lateralization is currently the surgery of choice for animals with severe clinical signs related to bilateral laryngeal paralysis.

Prognosis

Aspiration pneumonia is the most common complication following arytenoid lateralization and can be seen in 20–30% of patients. It may occur immediately postoperatively or up to 3 years after surgery. Factors significantly associated with a higher risk of developing aspiration pneumonia include preoperative aspiration pneumonia, esophageal disease, temporary tracheostomy placement, and concurrent neoplastic disease (MacPhail and Monnet 2001). However, most dogs survive postoperative aspiration pneumonia with appropriate therapy, and owners are ultimately pleased with the clinical outcome. Other complications following surgical treatment of laryngeal paralysis include suture failure leading to acute upper airway obstruction and incisional seroma.

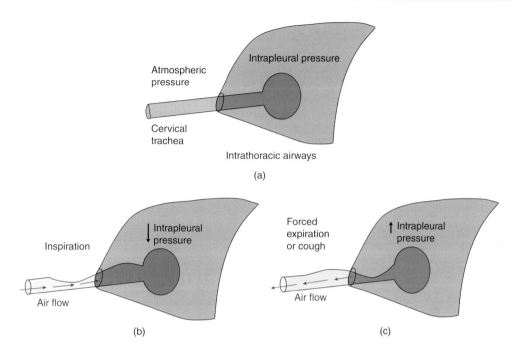

Figure 5.3. The airways are exposed to atmospheric pressure in the cervical region and intrapleural pressure in the intrathorac region (a). During inspiration, intrapleural pressure drops to create a pressure gradient that results in flow of air from the mouth to the alveolus. The dog with weakened cartilage rings in the cervical region experiences collapse on inspiration (b). During a forced expiration or cough, intrapleural pressure becomes positive and the pressure gradient across the airways favors collapse in the intrathoracic region when cartilage is weak (c). (Modified from *Waltham Focus* 11(2): 3–8, 2001, with permission.)

Tracheal/Airway Collapse

Pathophysiology

The etiology of tracheal collapse is unknown, but some dogs have been shown to have a reduction in chondrocytes and lack of glycosaminoglycan and chondroitin sulfate in tracheal cartilage. This leads to weakening of cartilage with flattening of the tracheal rings. Typically, tracheal collapse is in a dorsoventral direction with prolapse of an elongated dorsal tracheal membrane into the lumen of the airway. This dynamic collapse leads to mechanical irritation of the opposing mucosa, which enhances tracheal edema and inflammation. The mucociliary apparatus is disrupted and there is increased risk for small airway disease or mucus trapping. The cervical trachea collapses during inspiration while the intrathoracic portion of the trachea collapses on expiration because of the pressure gradients that develop during the respiratory cycle (Figure 5.3). Many dogs with tracheal collapse have collapse of both the cervical and intrathoracic trachea. In some dogs, the principal bronchi also are collapsed, with the right middle and left cranial lobar bronchi affected most commonly. When bronchial collapse is found in conjunction with tracheal collapse, this is termed tracheobronchomalacia. In some dogs, only lobar or lower airway collapse is detected and this is termed bronchomalacia. Chronic bronchitis can be found in conjunction with tracheal collapse or bronchomalacia.

History

Tracheal collapse is seen most commonly in small or toy-breed dogs, such as the Yorkshire terrier, Pomeranian, Poodle, Maltese, and Chihuahua, while bronchomalacia can be seen in small- and medium-sized dogs. Tracheal collapse is diagnosed rarely in large-breed dogs and in cats, although large-breed dogs may be affected by bronchial collapse. The condition is less common in the cat, although tracheobronchial collapse may accompany chronic bronchial disease. At the time of presentation, dogs can range from 1 to 15 years of age, depending on the degree of airway collapse and the presence of contributing clinical conditions. Dogs are commonly overweight, and both sexes are equally affected.

Most dogs with tracheal collapse have a chronic history of waxing and waning respiratory difficulty or cough that has grown progressively worse over time or has become refractory to treatment. Exacerbation of cough after eating and drinking or with excitement is common in dogs with tracheal collapse. The cough may be described as paroxysmal, dry, or as a "honking" cough. Owners may mistake the cough for vomiting or will report gagging or retching in association with the cough as the animal attempts to clear secretions from the airways. Worsened tachypnea, exercise intolerance, and respiratory distress tend to occur during physical exertion, with heat stress, or in humid conditions. This may be the result of airway collapse alone, chronic bronchitis, infectious airway disease, and/or concurrent upper airway obstruction (edema, saccular eversion, or laryngeal paralysis). Cyanosis or syncope occurs in severely affected animals due to complete airway obstruction, vagally mediated syncope, or pulmonary hypertension.

Physical examination

Dogs with airway collapse are usually systemically healthy and they are often overweight. The respiratory pattern can appear normal at rest, while marked expiratory effort can indicate bronchial collapse or concurrent bronchitis. Auscultation over the trachea can reveal musical or wheezing sounds caused by turbulent airflow through the narrowed lumen. Dramatic stridor over the upper airway is suggestive of concurrent laryngeal paresis or paralysis, which has been reported in up to 30% of dogs with tracheal collapse. Inspiratory and expiratory stridor can also be heard in dogs with severe tracheal collapse that results in a narrowed and fixed tracheal diameter. A flattened cervical trachea can be palpated in severe tracheal collapse. Most dogs with tracheal or airway collapse have a readily induced cough. Caution is warranted when palpating the trachea in dogs with reports of severe coughing because it may induce a life-threatening crisis of coughing or cough syncope.

Lung sounds can be difficult to assess in dogs with tracheal or airway collapse due to tachypnea, obesity, or referred upper airway sounds. Crackles associated with mucus plugging and airway closure can sometimes be auscultated when concurrent chronic bronchitis or bronchomalacia is present. Careful cardiac auscultation should be performed because 20% or more of middle-aged, small-breed dogs have mitral valve insufficiency in addition to airway collapse. Hepatomegaly is a common finding in dogs with tracheal collapse and may be related to fatty infiltration or a nonspecific hepatopathy.

Diagnostic findings

Although the diagnosis of tracheal collapse can be strongly presumed based on the signalment, history, and physical examination findings, a complete diagnostic work-up should be performed to define concurrent disorders and provide appropriate therapy. Routine hematologic testing may detect predisposing conditions or concurrent disease in dogs with tracheal collapse. Increased liver enzymes are not uncommon in dogs with airway collapse, and elevations in serum bile acids have also been reported, although the cause for this is unclear (Bauer et al. 2006).

Radiographs are essential both to examine airway diameter and to detect concurrent pulmonary or cardiac disorders. Cautious interpretation of the cardiac silhouette is warranted in obese dogs. Fat around the pericardial space and reduced lung volume can lead to the false impression of cardiomegaly. However, right-sided heart enlargement may be present in dogs with severe tracheal collapse, pulmonary disease, or other factors that predispose to the development of pulmonary hypertension.

It is important to note that airway collapse is a dynamic process and radiographs often give a false impression of the presence or absence of collapse. In the cervical region, overlying structures such as the esophagus and neck muscles can obscure details. Evaluation of left and right lateral views may improve distinction of structures; however, differences in positioning and in the phase of respiration may make it difficult to compare these views directly. Obtaining inspiratory and expiratory phases of respiration can be helpful because the cervical region should collapse on inspiration while the intrathoracic airways should collapse on expiration; however, the difficulty in timing these radiographs precisely limits the actual value. In comparison to fluoroscopy, radiographs underestimate the severity of tracheal collapse and are less able to detect intrathoracic airway collapse, which is often more severe than cervical collapse (Macready et al. 2007) (Figure 5.4). Therefore, while radiographs are useful as a screening tool for collapsing airways, they cannot be relied on for the diagnosis and likely will provide inaccurate information regarding the location and severity of tracheobronchial collapse. Fluoroscopy, where available, is beneficial in providing information on the degree of dynamic airway obstruction, and it also allows correlation of airway collapse with cardiac and respiratory cycles. Additional findings such as cranial lung herniation during cough can be detected (Figure 5.5).

Bronchoscopy can document tracheal collapse when radiographs or fluoroscopy is inconclusive and is useful for grading the degree of collapse (Figure 5.6). In addition, bronchoscopy readily identifies bronchomalacia, which can be static or dynamic (Figure 5.7). Bronchoalveolar lavage or an endotracheal wash sample can be used to document bacterial or *Mycoplasma* infection and to detect inflammation by cytologic examination, although bacteria are rarely involved in tracheal collapse and bronchomalacia. The risk of anesthesia for bronchoscopy can be significant in dogs with airway collapse, especially in obese

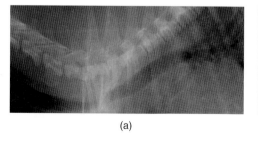
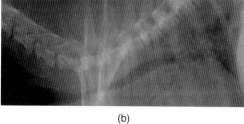

(a) (b)

Figure 5.4. Inspiratory (a) and expiratory (b) fluoroscopic images from a 13-year-old MC Terrier mix with intrathoracic airway collapse. Note the dramatic reduction in the diameter of the intrathoracic trachea and carina, and the loss of air column within principal and lobar bronchi in (b).

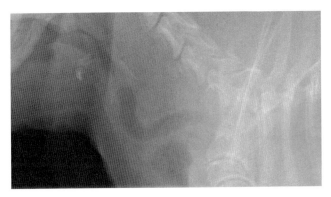

Figure 5.5. Fluoroscopic image from a 15-year-old FS Pug demonstrates dramatic ventral deviation of the cervical trachea and cranial herniation of the lung through the thoracic inlet during a cough.

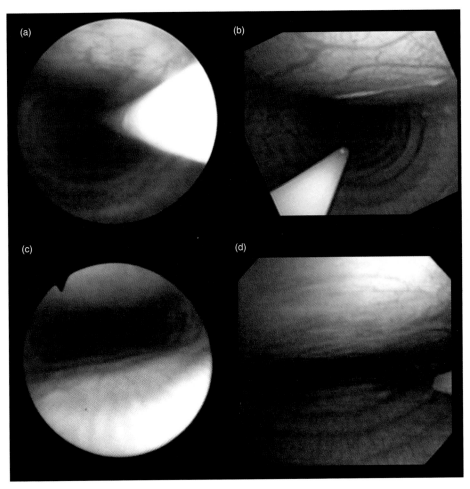

Figure 5.6. Grade I: The cartilage ring structure of the trachea remains circular and is almost normal. Slight protrusion of the dorsal tracheal membrane into the lumen reduces the diameter by <25% (a). Grade II: Flattening of the tracheal cartilage leads to lengthening of the dorsal tracheal membrane and further reduces the luminal diameter to approximately 50% (b). Grade III: The tracheal cartilage rings are severely flattened and the trachealis muscle contacts the inner surface of the tracheal cartilage. The lumen is reduced by 75% (c). Grade IV: The trachealis muscle is collapsed onto the inner surface of the cartilage, leading to complete obstruction of the lumen. A double lumen may be seen in some cases (d).

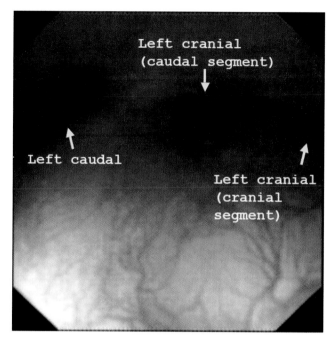

Figure 5.7. Bronchoscopic image demonstrating 70–100% collapse of lobar bronchi to the left lung lobe.

animals with severe tracheal sensitivity or in hyperexcitable dogs. A slow recovery from anesthesia is advisable to minimize stress, and an oxygen-enriched environment should be available. One milliliter of 1% lidocaine sprayed into the distal trachea at the end of bronchoscopy can help decrease the cough reflex.

Treatment

Animals that have marked respiratory difficulty and coughing may require inpatient management. Stress should be minimized, and oxygen supplementation can be beneficial. Cough suppression and sedation can be achieved with butorphanol (0.05–0.1 mg/kg SC q4–6 hours), and addition of acepromazine (0.01–0.1 mg/kg SC) can have a synergistic effect in producing sedation. Caution should be employed when using the drugs together to avoid oversedation that might require intubation. To decrease laryngeal or tracheal inflammation, a single dose of dexamethasone-SP (0.10–0.25 mg/kg i.v.) or prednisolone sodium succinate (15–30 mg/kg i.v.) can be administered.

Outpatient management should be designed to treat disorders identified in the diagnostic work-up. If the dog is not stable for collection of an airway sample or if cultures are pending, a trial on doxycycline (3–5 mg/kg PO BID) can be employed to treat potential *Mycoplasma* infection and to provide mild anti-inflammatory effects. Bronchodilators may help reduce cough in animals with bronchomalacia by decreasing the tendency of intrathoracic airway to collapse. Suggested drugs include sustained release theophylline (5–10 mg/kg PO BID), terbutaline (0.625–5 mg/dog PO BID–TID), and albuterol syrup (50 µg/kg PO TID). Airway infection is treated with appropriate antibiotics as determined by airway sampling. If chronic bronchitis is diagnosed, corticosteroids should be employed (see later in this

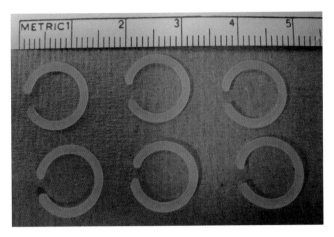

Figure 5.8. Tracheal rings used for external support in dogs with cervical tracheal collapse.

chapter). If marked tracheal inflammation is noted, a short course (5–7 days) of prednisone can be beneficial, although inhaled corticosteroids are preferred because they have limited side effects such as weight gain and panting that can exacerbate airway collapse. Finally, narcotic cough suppressants are often required to control cough and should be administered often enough to control cough without inducing severe sedation. Suggested drugs include hydrocodone (0.22 mg/kg PO BID–QID) and butorphanol (0.55 mg/kg PO BID–QID). Starting with a frequent dosing interval and gradually extending the time between doses and/or reducing the dose appears to be most effective in controlling signs and avoiding the development of tolerance.

Ancillary measures include avoidance of collars and decreased exposure to heat and humidity. Encouraging weight loss in obese animals is essential. This intervention alone can result in a significant reduction in cough and improvement in overall health. Upper airway surgery, if needed, can also reduce clinical signs. Dogs that fail medical management require additional intervention. In dogs with cervical tracheal collapse, placement of tracheal ring prostheses (Figure 5.8) will result in dramatic reduction in clinical signs (Buback et al. 1996). The primary complication of surgery is development of laryngeal paralysis from damage to the recurrent laryngeal nerve during or after surgery. When intrathoracic tracheal collapse is detected, placement of an intraluminal stenting device (Figure 5.9) can be successful in reducing clinical signs (Moritz et al. 2004, Sura et al. 2008). It is critical that the appropriate

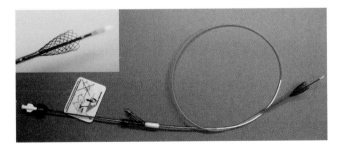

Figure 5.9. Catheter delivery system and close-up of a distal deployment stent manufactured for intraluminal support of intrathoracic or complete tracheal collapse. (Courtesy of Infiniti Medical, www.infinitimedical.com.)

type and size of stent are used to attain a successful outcome (Weisse 2009). Complications of stent placement include migration, granuloma formation, or breakage of the stent.

Prognosis

Tracheal collapse with or without airway collapse is a common cause of cough in small-breed dogs. Bronchomalacia is found frequently in large-breed dogs also: however, because it requires bronchoscopy for identification, the condition is underdiagnosed. Most animals can be managed successfully with an individualized treatment plan directed against the abnormalities noted during diagnostic testing; however, the underlying pathology of airway collapse is irreversible. Recurrent clinical signs should be anticipated and for dogs that are refractory to therapy, more aggressive intervention should be investigated.

Bronchiectasis

Pathophysiology

Bronchiectasis is described as irreversible dilatation of the bronchi with accumulation of suppurative airway secretions. The disorder is a poorly characterized condition associated with chronic obstructive, inflammatory, or infectious airway diseases in dogs and cats. In the dog, foreign body pneumonia, ciliary dyskinesia, smoke inhalation, chronic aspiration pneumonia, eosinophilic bronchopneumopathy, or chronic bronchitis can lead to the development of bronchiectasis. In the cat, bronchiectasis has been recognized in association with chronic inflammatory airway disease, and the radiographic appearance can be similar to that seen with cystic bronchogenic carcinoma.

History and signalment

Dogs or cats that have bronchiectasis as part of the syndrome of primary ciliary dyskinesia are typically young on presentation and have a chronic history of serous to mucoid nasal secretions and cough that responds to antibiotics but recurs (see Chapter 6).

Animals with acquired bronchiectasis are middle aged to older and have a chronic cough or recurrent pneumonia. Disease is clinically recognized more often in dogs than cats, and Cocker Spaniels are predisposed to the disorder.

Physical examination

There are no specific physical examination features that characterize bronchiectasis. A rapid shallow breathing pattern and abnormal thoracic auscultation may be present in animals with concurrent pneumonia; however, some affected dogs may display only tracheal sensitivity associated with airway inflammation. A moist cough is often induced.

Diagnostic findings

Definitive diagnosis of bronchiectasis is difficult in veterinary medicine because early radiographic lesions are subtle, and dilated, thickened airways are not readily detectable, particularly if pneumonia is absent. When visible radiographically, disease should be considered

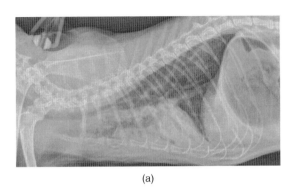
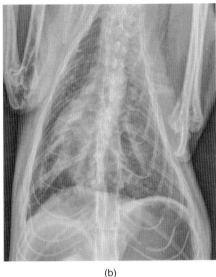

(a)   (b)

Figure 5.10.   Right lateral (a) and dorsoventral (b) radiographs from a 10-year-old FS DLH with radiographically apparent bronchiectasis involving the left cranial lung lobe (cranial and caudal segments). A pneumonic infiltrate in the left cranial lung lobe outlines the bronchi and a diffuse bronchial pattern is present throughout the remainder of the lung fields.

advanced and irreversible (Figure 5.10). Computed tomography (CT) is used for recognition of dilated airways in human medicine but has only recently been used to aid in the diagnosis of pulmonary disorders in veterinary medicine (Figure 5.11). Visualization of the airways through bronchoscopy allows documentation of bronchiectasis; however, the operator must have knowledge of normal airway anatomy to recognize the abnormality. With bronchiectasis, the normal rounded bifurcations at bronchial branch points are replaced by dilated and more oval or irregular appearing airway openings (Figure 5.12). Airway space is increased as airways are pulled open by the reduction in supporting parenchyma.

During bronchoscopy or by use of a tracheal wash, airway samples should be collected in affected dogs for cytology and aerobic, anaerobic, and *Mycoplasma* cultures. Cytology is generally characterized by a high proportion of nondegenerate or degenerate neutrophils. Given the purulence of secretions and the antibiotic responsiveness of many patients, deep-seated pulmonary infection likely contributes to the disease process, even though bacteria are not always detected on culture.

Young animals diagnosed with bronchiectasis should be evaluated for primary ciliary dyskinesia (see Chapter 6).

Treatment

In dogs with neutrophilic airway cytology, long-term, broad-spectrum antibiotics are indicated for control of clinical signs, prevention of worsening airway pathology, and avoidance of systemic manifestations of chronic disease such as anemia or glomerulonephritis. Drugs that penetrate the pulmonary tissue well should be employed, such as doxycycline, azithromycin, enrofloxacin, trimethoprim-sulfa, chloramphenicol, and

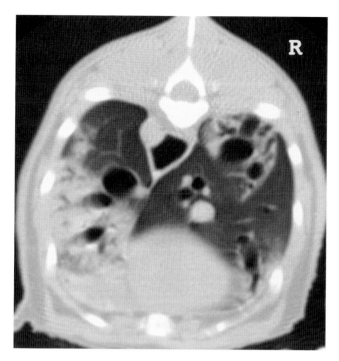

Figure 5.11. Computed tomography image from the cat depicted in Figure 5.10 reveals marked dilation of all airways with lack of normal tapering into the periphery. Alveolar infiltrates are noted in the left lung lobe.

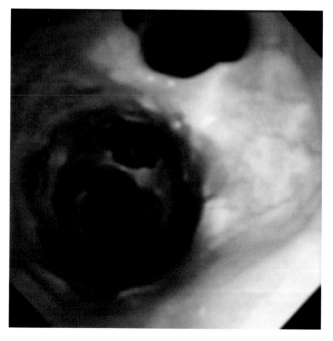

Figure 5.12. Bronchoscopic image of the lungs from the cat in Figures 5.10 and 5.11. Airways are dilated, the epithelial surface is hyperemic, and mucosal nodules are evident.

clindamycin. Six weeks to six months of treatment with one antibiotic or a rotation of antibiotics monthly may be required to control pulmonary inflammation. In severe cases, life-long antibiotics should be considered. Focal bronchiectasis is amenable to surgical resection of affected lung lobes. Dogs with bronchiectasis associated with eosinophilic lung disease are treated as described in Chapter 6. With all forms of bronchiectasis, cough suppressants must be avoided. Saline nebulization followed by coupage can help liquefy and loosen airway secretions, and *N*-acetylcysteine may be beneficial (see Chapter 3).

Disease in cats is more challenging to treat because bacteria are almost never isolated and cats do not seem to respond to antibiotics as well as dogs often will. Inhaled corticosteroids can be helpful in improving respirations unless inspissated airway secretions prevent penetration of the drug to the mucosa. Ancillary management with nebulization can be valuable.

Prognosis

Dogs with bronchiectasis can suffer recurrent bouts of life-threatening bacterial pneumonia and may develop secondary diseases such as glomerulonephritis associated with chronic antigenic stimulus. Continual antibiotic treatment and respiratory therapy are required for some dogs, while others may have periodic episodes of antibiotic–responsive pneumonia interspersed with long stages of normal health. Similarly, prognosis for dogs with ciliary dyskinesia and bronchiectasis is variable. Some dogs are only mildly affected throughout life or become subclinical as they age, while others may succumb to pneumonia.

Infectious Diseases

Canine Infectious Respiratory Disease Complex ("Kennel Cough")

Pathophysiology

Canine infectious respiratory disease (CIRD) complex is associated with multiple pathogens, including parainfluenza virus (CPIV), canine adenovirus (CAV-2), and canine distemper virus (CDV), as well as the newly recognized canine viruses respiratory coronavirus (CRCoV), canine herpesvirus (CHV-1), and canine influenza virus (CIV). Viral infection of epithelial cells damages cells and alters local immunity, which predisposes the animal to infection with both primary respiratory pathogens (*Bordetella* and *Mycoplasma*) and other commensal and pathogenic bacteria. Infection is prevalent in animals that are housed in shelter environments or held in close confinement because the viruses are highly contagious and easily spread by aerosolization or fomites.

History and signalment

Clinical signs of nasal discharge and/or cough are usually seen 2–10 days postexposure to an infected animal and the dose of pathogens encountered may play a role in virulence and the severity of clinical disease. Young animals in shelters are quickly exposed to most organisms and will readily spread the disease to animals of any age in the general population. While infection with viral organisms usually results in a mild cough, infection with *Bordetella* classically results in a dry, paroxysmal, "seal bark" cough. Infection with canine herpesvirus tends to result in ocular involvement with marked conjunctivitis and blepharospasm as well as respiratory signs. Viral infections are typically self-limiting, with resolution of signs in 7–10 days, although *Bordetella* and canine influenza virus infections can result in chronic cough that requires specific investigation and treatment.

Physical examination

Most dogs with CIRD remain systemically healthy although neonates and immune-compromised patients are susceptible to development of pneumonia. Most dogs display obvious tracheal sensitivity but have a normal respiratory pattern and normal lung sounds unless bronchopneumonia develops. Increasing severity of disease is recognized by the development of tachypnea, harsh lung sounds, fever, and lethargy. With development of bacterial infection, a moist and productive cough can develop, and crackles or wheezes may be auscultated. Physical examination abnormalities are usually confined to the respiratory tract, although CHV-1 can cause surface ocular disease, and retinochoroiditis can be detected in dogs with CDV.

Diagnostic findings

In privately owned pet animals that are systemically healthy, the diagnosis of CIRD is usually based on history and clinical signs. In an outbreak situation or in an ill animal, it is important to identify the infecting organism(s) to limit spread of disease and provide appropriate treatment. A CBC may show changes in lymphocyte numbers suggestive of a viral insult or alterations in neutrophils due to bacterial infection. If marked conjunctivitis or blepharospasm is noted, a fluorescein stain should be applied to the eyes and may detect the classic dendritic ulcer of CHV-1. Thoracic radiographs would be expected to show a diffuse interstitial infiltrate in viral pneumonia and alveolar infiltrates in the presence of bacterial infection.

In animals with primarily upper respiratory tract signs, a nasal, ocular, or pharyngeal swab can be assessed for organisms through culture or molecular assay. It is important to note that these tests can confirm the presence of an organism but do not prove causation of disease. Limitations of these assays must also be considered. For example, canine respiratory coronavirus is difficult to culture and molecular identification or serology is usually required. The timing of viral shedding in relationship to the onset of clinical signs alters the value of viral culture. Experimental CHV-1 infection in dogs results in peak ocular manifestations of disease by day 7–10 yet viral shedding peaks at day 5 and declines substantially by day 10 (Ledbetter et al. 2009). In the case of CIV, diagnosis based on virus isolation is also problematic. Clinical signs begin 2–3 days postinfection but the virus is shed only for a maximum of 5–7 days, making it unlikely that culture or PCR will detect virus unless the dog is presented very early in the course of disease. Documentation of CIV infection (or exposure to CIV) is best made through assessment of hemagglutination inhibition serum titers for virus-specific antibodies. When possible, acute and convalescent serum samples (preferably 14 days after clinical signs are detected) should be evaluated to detect more than fourfold increase in titer. Usually only convalescent serum is available but because vaccination for CIV is not widespread, a positive titer indicates that the dog has been exposed to the virus (Crawford et al. 2005). Acute and convalescent serum samples can also be useful in the diagnosis of CPIV and CAV-2, although testing is not usually performed because dogs fully recover from infection and vaccinal titers can confuse interpretation.

If an animal with evidence of lower respiratory tract involvement in CIRD is stable for anesthesia, collection of airway samples would be recommended for virus isolation, bacterial cultures (aerobic, anaerobic, and *Mycoplasma*), cytology with immunocytochemistry or immunofluorescence, and PCR.

Treatment

In uncomplicated cases, supportive care results in resolution of signs. Physical activity is restricted, collars are avoided, and nutrition and hydration are supported. If bacterial infection is considered unlikely, cough suppressants can be used to break the cycle of repetitive airway injury; however, there is a risk for development of pneumonia if bacteria are trapped in the lungs. Many dogs are initially treated with antibiotics for secondary infection. Doxycycline and chloramphenicol are reasonable antibiotics to use because of their efficacy against *Mycoplasma* species. *Bordetella* has in vitro susceptibility to a number of antibiotics but may not be sensitive in vivo because the organism infects cilia, which are not readily penetrated by systemically administered agents. Nebulization of an aminoglycoside may be required to reduce bacterial numbers. Specific antiviral therapy is not currently available or recommended for affected dogs.

Prognosis

Most dogs that become infected with organisms involved with CIRD survive, although fatalities can be seen, particularly with distemper virus and influenza virus. CIV and *Bordetella* infections can result in chronic signs. Subclinical shedders represent a source of environmental exposure for susceptible dogs.

In a dense population of dogs, appropriate infection control measures should be in place to limit spread of respiratory disease. Reducing crowding, improving air exchanges, and using rigorous hygiene practices are all helpful. Most viruses are readily destroyed by bleach, and workers should be alert for the possibility of spreading disease while working among animals. When disease is detected in a population, limiting contact of susceptible dogs with those showing clinical signs is important; however, dogs can spread infection in the absence of clinical signs. Ideally, sick dogs should be kept completely isolated from the rest of the population, and full clothing coverage, gloves, and booties should be used in environments containing sick animals. New dogs that enter the environment should be held in isolation until the incubation period ($\sim$7–10 days) for infectious diseases has passed.

Vaccination against the commonly encountered pathogens reduces but does not eliminate clinical disease. The 2006 AAHA Canine Vaccination Guidelines recommend vaccination against distemper, parvovirus, canine adenovirus-2, and rabies, and routine vaccination against the upper respiratory tract viruses should help limit secondary bacterial involvement. Noncore vaccines should also be considered in select instances. Use of the monovalent intranasal vaccine for *Bordetella* can be used in susceptible dogs that will be exposed to a dense population of dogs because it provides protection within just 72 hours of administration. Vaccination in the face of an outbreak has not appreciably lessened clinical disease. Conditional license has been granted for a vaccine against canine influenza virus (Intervet/ Schering Plough Animal Health, Elkhorn, NE) due to the vaccine's ability to decrease the duration of coughing, reduce viral shedding, and diminish pulmonary lesions induced by the virus (June 2009). The vaccine is produced from killed virus and will result in seroconversion. Therefore, risk factors for disease must be considered when deciding whether to vaccinate patients against the influenza virus.

Parasitic Bronchitis

Pathophysiology

Parasites implicated in respiratory disease include lungworms *Filaroides hirthi* (canine), *Aelurostrongylus abstrusus* (feline), *Capillaria aerophila* (dogs and cats), *Oslerus osleri* (canine), *Paragonimus kellicotti* (dogs and cats), and larval migration of *Toxocara, Ancylostoma,* or *Strongyloides*. Specific features of life cycle, transmission, and diagnosis of each parasite are summarized in Table 5.2.

History and signalment

Parasitic bronchitis occurs more commonly in young outdoor animals and particularly those that hunt. However, it may be encountered in any large- or small-breed dog regardless of activity because the mechanism for transmission of many of these parasites is incompletely understood. Most airway parasites are associated with cough; however, *O. osleri* and *Paragonimus* can lead to difficulty breathing. With infection by *Oslerus*, this is due to obstruction of the trachea by parasitic nodules while *Paragonimus* leads to difficulty breathing when rupture of a parasitic cyst results in pneumothorax.

Physical examination

Tracheal sensitivity is generally present with most parasitic infections, and wheezing may be heard because of airway inflammation or obstruction. Infection by *Paragonimus* and resultant pneumothorax can be detected by the presence of tachypnea and an absence of breath sounds dorsally due to air accumulation. Percussion can detect hyper-resonance in the dorsal thorax.

Diagnostic findings

Blood work may reveal eosinophilia and fecal examinations can be diagnostic (Table 5.2) although because parasites are shed intermittently, a negative fecal does not rule out infection. *Filaroides, Capillaria,* and *Aelurostrongylus* can result in nodular or miliary interstitial densities or in a bronchial pattern. Radiographic infiltrates are concentrated in the caudal lobes in patients with larval migration. *O. osleri* results in nodules within the trachea near the carina. These can be seen radiographically or during bronchosopy and appear as round, soft tissue densities. Parasitic larvae can be found in biopsy samples or in bronchoalveolar lavage fluid cytology. *Paragonimus* forms nodular densities or either air- or fluid-filled cysts. Pneumothorax is evident radiographically as loss of vascular and bronchial markings in the periphery (see Chapter 7).

Table 5.2. Clinical characteristics, diagnostic methods, and treatment for parasitic bronchitis

Parasite	Method of Transmission	Special Features	Clinical Findings	Diagnosis	Treatment
Filaroides hirthi	Fecal–oral	Young dogs in confinement or kennels	Cough	L1 in feces (Baermann)	Ivermectin (1 mg/kg once weekly × 2 Albendazole (50 mg/kg BID for 5 days) Fenbendazole 50 mg/kg/day for 3 weeks
Aelurostrongylus abstrusus	Ingestion of intermediate host (snail, bird, or rodent)	Outdoor cats or hunters	Cough	L1 in feces (Baermann) or tracheal wash	Fenbendazole 50 mg/kg daily for 10 days
Capillaria aerophila	Ingestion of eggs or intermediate host (earthworm)			Eggs in fecal float (whipworm-like)	Fenbendazole 50 mg/kg daily for 10 days Ivermectin 0.2–0.2 µg/kg SQ for 1–2 dosed
Oslerus osleri	Regurgitative feeding	Dogs exposed to wild canids?	Obstructive respirations, cough	Nodules at carina	Unknown
Paragonimus kellicotti	Ingestion of crayfish	Hunters	Cough, tachypnea, pneumothorax	Large operculated egg in tracheal wash or feces (sedimentation or zinc sulphate centrifugation flotation)	Praziquantel 25 mg/kg PO TID for 2–3 days Fenbendazole 50 mg/kg PO for 10–14 days
Larval migration	Perinatal	Young animals	Cough, tachypnea	Fecal flotation for ascarid eggs, eosinophilic airway wash	Fenbendazole 50 mg/kg daily for 10 days

Treatment

Most airway parasites can be treated with fenbendazole or ivermectin although *O. osleri* can be particularly refractory to therapy. When rupture of a Paragonimus cyst is identified, a chest tap is required to alleviate respiratory difficulty and lung lobectomy is usually required.

Prognosis

Most animals will recover from parasitic bronchitis. Mortality can occur with rupture of *Paragonimus* cysts or because of airway obstruction associated with refractory infection by *O. olseri*.

Inflammatory Disorders

Inflammatory Laryngitis

Pathophysiology

Nonspecific inflammation of the larynx is common secondary to any infectious or inflammatory disease of the lower airway, and can also be encountered in animals with vomiting disorders due to acid injury to the upper airway. It can also occur secondary to trauma associated with choke chain injury, an insect bite, or inhalation of noxious fumes. Less commonly, primary inflammation of the larynx is encountered. In the cat, this lesion can appear similar to a neoplasm and biopsy differentiation is crucial. The etiology of inflammation is usually not determined in these cases.

History and signalment

Animals with primary or secondary laryngitis can be of any age or breed. Owner complaints are similar to those seen with other laryngeal diseases and include inspiratory difficulty, dysphonia, inappetance or difficulty swallowing, and retching.

Physical examination

Stridor or loud inspiratory sounds over the larynx are common, and cervical palpation may reveal an unusual larynx (firm or asymmetric) in some dogs or cats.

Diagnostic findings

Cervical radiographs may reveal increased soft tissue density in the region of the larynx or caudal retraction of the laryngeal apparatus (Figure 5.1). Visual inspection and biopsy of the larynx are required for full evaluation. Secondary laryngitis is associated with hyperemia and mucosal edema, while primary or granulomatous laryngitis is typically associated with a mass effect on the larynx. A tissue sample for histopathology can be acquired using 2- or 3-mm cup biopsy forceps (Sontec Instruments, Centennial, CO, or Karl Storz

Veterinary Endoscopy, Goleta, CA), and will generally reveal lymphocytic or granulomatous inflammation.

Treatment

Secondary laryngitis will usually resolve with treatment of the underling airway or gastrointestinal condition. Primary inflammatory laryngitis may require debulking surgery, laryngectomy, and/or tracheostomy to alleviate respiratory distress. Some cases respond adequately to glucocorticoids alone or in combination with surgery (Tasker et al. 1999).

Canine Chronic Bronchitis

Pathophysiology

Chronic bronchitis is defined by the presence of a daily cough that occurs for at least 2 months of the year and lacks a specific cause. Cough is related to activation of irritant receptors in the airways by products of inflammatory cells. Recruitment of inflammatory cells may occur by exposure to environmental pollutants, second-hand smoke, or inhaled irritants. Usually the etiology is unknown. Neutrophilic infiltration of the airway results in release of proteases, elastases, and oxidizing products that perpetuate inflammation and airway damage. Histologic examination of mucosal biopsy specimens from dogs with chronic bronchitis reveals hypertrophy and hyperplasia of mucous glands and goblet cells, fibrosis of the lamina propria, and epithelial erosion with squamous metaplasia. These changes contribute to obstruction of airflow through accumulation of mucus within the airway and lead to clinical signs of cough and exercise intolerance. Focal or generalized bronchomalacia can sometimes accompany chronic bronchitis, perhaps because inflammatory mediators lead to weakening of cartilage or have effects on airway smooth muscle tone.

History and signalment

Chronic bronchitis is a disease of middle-aged to older dogs, and both large- and small-breed dogs are affected. The predominant clinical complaint is persistent coughing, which may be a dry hacking cough or moist and productive when copious amounts of respiratory secretions are produced. A "goose honk" cough may predominate in small-breed dogs that have concurrent tracheal or airway collapse. Dogs are typically healthy and relatively active, although in the later stages of disease, exercise intolerance or heavy breathing can be reported. Severely affected animals may experience intermittent cyanosis or collapse.

Physical examination

Dogs with chronic bronchitis are often overweight but appear otherwise healthy. Some dogs will pant excessively while dogs severely affected by bronchitis can have prolonged expiration or an expiratory push. Tracheal sensitivity is usually present because of nonspecific airway inflammation. Thoracic auscultation can be normal or may reveal coarse, diffuse crackles associated with mucus accumulation or small airway collapse. Expiratory wheezes are considered the hallmark of chronic bronchitis but are not always present. Large airway collapse should be suspected when a snapping sound is auscultated over the thoracic

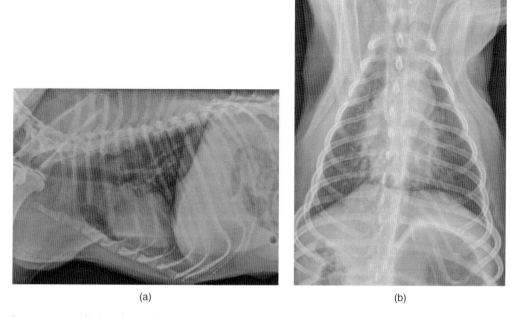

(a)   (b)

Figure 5.13.   Right lateral (a) and dorsoventral (b) radiographs from 12-year-old MC Basenji with a 2-year history of cough. Bronchial walls are thickened and easily visualized on both views. Spondylosis of the thoracic spine is also evident.

cage during expiration. Careful cardiac auscultation is advised to detect concurrent valvular insufficiency, which is common in older small-breed dogs.

Diagnostic findings

The diagnosis of chronic bronchitis is one of exclusion because infectious bronchitis (*Mycoplasma* or *Bordetella*) and airway collapse cause similar historical and physical examination findings. Clinicopathologic abnormalities are typically absent in dogs with chronic bronchitis. Arterial blood gas analysis (if performed) generally shows only mild-to-moderate hypoxemia, and hypercarbia is not detected until late in the disease if respiratory failure ensues.

Thoracic radiography is an important part of the diagnostic work-up to confirm the likelihood of chronic bronchitis and to rule out other conditions. Classically, a generalized increase in interstitial or bronchial infiltrates is expected in dogs with chronic bronchitis. End-on bronchi (doughnuts) and airways seen in longitudinal section (tram lines) represent airway walls thickened by inflammation (Figure 5.13). However, radiographs are insensitive for detecting chronic bronchitis, and in a case-controlled evaluation, only increased thickness of airway walls and increased numbers of visible airway walls differed between normal dogs and dogs with bronchitis (Mantis et al. 1998). Importantly, normal chest radiographs do not rule out the diagnosis of chronic bronchitis.

Collecting airway samples by tracheal wash or bronchoscopy is recommended to characterize the cellular infiltrate in the airway and to rule out infectious causes of cough. Bronchoscopy is particularly useful when typical radiographic findings of bronchitis are

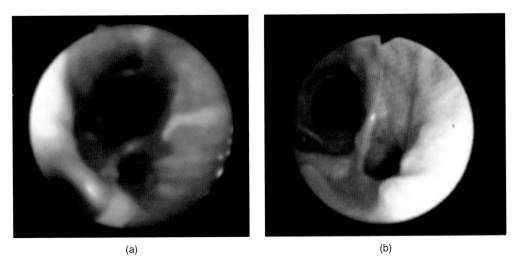

(a)   (b)

Figure 5.14. Bronchoscopic images from two dogs with chronic bronchitis. The mucosa is dramatically hyperemic and thick mucus is evident streaming from the airways (a). The mucosa is mildly hyperemic, and nodular proliferations are present that distort the epithelial surface (b).

lacking; however, careful case selection is important to avoid complications. Obese dogs with marked expiratory effort seem more likely to have anesthetic difficulties, and judicious therapeutic trials might be considered for these dogs. Dogs with chronic bronchitis have airway hyperemia, the airway mucosa has a cobblestone or irregular appearance, and most dogs have increased mucus lining the airway (Figure 5.14). In animals with long-standing bronchitis, fibrotic inflammatory nodules can be seen protruding into the bronchial lumen.

Chronic bronchitis can be confirmed with airway sampling via tracheal wash or bronchoscopy. Cytologically, chronic bronchitis is characterized by an increase in total cell numbers and a predominance of nondegenerate neutrophils (Figure 5.15). Some dogs have a high proportion of eosinophils in airway washings or mixed inflammation, although the significance of this type of inflammatory response is unknown. Increased mucus is present in many airway samples, and Curschmann's spirals (bronchial casts of airway mucus) are sometimes noted. Epithelial cells and squamous metaplasia may also be seen on cytologic examination.

Although suppurative inflammation is present on cytologic examination, bacterial infection is not a significant problem in the majority of dogs with chronic bronchitis. A light growth of bacteria is not unexpected because the trachea and large airways of dogs are not always sterile (Peeters et al. 2000). Because *Mycoplasma* is part of the normal oral flora but can exacerbate lower airway injury, special culture techniques should be performed in bronchitic animals to rule out *Mycoplasma* infection.

Treatment

Anti-inflammatory agents
Therapy with glucocorticoids is successful in resolving clinical signs in the majority of dogs. It is essential that infectious diseases are ruled out before the initiation of anti-inflammatory treatment. Dosing of glucocorticoids should be tailored to the individual, with the severity

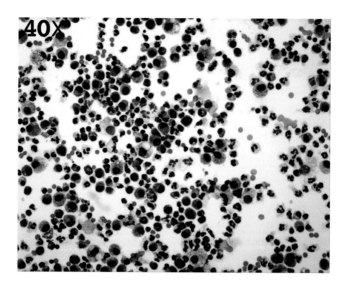

Figure 5.15. Neutrophilic airway cytology from a dog with chronic bronchitis (40×). In this cytospin preparation of bronchoalveolar lavage fluid, neutrophils represent 60% of the cell count, with the remainder of cells comprised of alveolar macrophages. Red blood cells suggest airway hemorrhage due to friability.

of clinical signs, chronicity of disease, and general systemic health considered in decisions regarding treatment. Short-acting steroids such as prednisone or prednisolone are generally safe and effective in dogs with uncomplicated bronchitis. In the early stages of disease, dogs often require dosages of glucocorticoids ranging from 0.5 to 1.0 mg/kg every 12 hours for 5–7 days to induce remission of clinical signs. As clinical signs abate, the dosage should be decreased by half every 5–10 days and, when possible, drugs should be administered on an alternate-day basis to allow normalization of the pituitary–adrenal axis. Long-term therapy (2–3 months) can be anticipated in most cases, although discontinuation of medication may be possible. When disease worsens in the early stages of treatment, a return to the higher dose of glucocorticoid that controlled clinical signs is generally required. Alternatively, treatment with inhaled steroids, bronchodilators, or antitussive agents can be added (see later). Long-acting glucocorticoids such as dexamethasone, triamcinolone, and methylprednisolone acetate are not recommended as they do not have a therapeutic advantage over prednisone and are associated with more severe derangements of the pituitary–adrenal axis.

To avoid most of the systemic effects of glucocorticoids, inhaled medications can be considered in animals that will tolerate administration via a facemask. See Chapter 3 for more details. Most dogs will require oral therapy with glucocorticoids for the first several weeks of therapy, but the oral dose can be tapered and discontinued more rapidly when inhaled medications are used concurrently. Some individuals may require lifelong or intermittent therapy with oral or inhaled corticosteroid.

Bronchodilators
Active bronchoconstriction is not a component of canine chronic bronchitis; however, bronchodilators can be clinically helpful in reducing cough or respiratory difficulty in dogs with bronchitis and they can allow a reduction in the dosage of glucocorticoid required to control clinical signs. Both methylxanthine derivatives and beta-agonists seem to act synergistically with glucocorticoids in the control of inflammatory lung disease. Bronchodilators may

provide other beneficial effects such as enhancing cardiac performance, reducing respiratory effort, and stimulating mucociliary clearance. In dogs that fail to respond adequately to glucocorticoids, a 2-week trial on a supplemental bronchodilator is a reasonable therapeutic option (see Chapter 3).

Antibiotics

Bacterial infection is not a component of chronic bronchitis; however, if a dog is not a good candidate for airway sampling, an antibiotic trial should be considered prior to instituting steroid therapy. Doxycycline is a reasonable antibiotic choice in this situation because of its efficacy against *Mycoplasma* and most other respiratory pathogens, as well as its anti-inflammatory effects.

Antitussive agents

Antitussives are most commonly required in dogs with chronic bronchitis that have concurrent airway collapse. When possible, use should be delayed until clinical response suggests that inflammation has resolved. See Chapter 3 for further details.

Additional therapy

Maximal efforts should be made to achieve weight loss in dogs with chronic bronchitis. Animals with concurrent tracheal collapse or marked tracheal sensitivity benefit from use of a harness in place of a collar. When stresses in the environment are encountered, such as cigarette smoke, pollutants, heat, or humidity, the animal should be removed to a cool, clean area.

Some dogs benefit from intermittent airway humidification via steam inhalation or nebulization to improve clearance of airway secretions. An ultrasonic nebulizer is preferred for respiratory therapy because it produces sufficiently small particles of saline (2–5 μm) to penetrate deep into the airways. Coupage of the chest or gentle exercise after nebulization facilitates clearance of secretions. For dogs with copious airway secretions, an oral mucolytic agent such as N-acetylcysteine might also be helpful (see Chapter 3).

Prognosis

When a diagnosis of chronic bronchitis is made, owners should understand that this is a chronic disease that can be controlled but never fully cured. The majority of animals have residual cough and exhibit clinical signs periodically throughout life. The presence of fibrosis and chronic inflammation on biopsy specimens confirms the irreversibility of airway disease. The goals of therapy are to control inflammation, thus limiting clinical signs, to diagnose and treat infection if it occurs, and to prevent worsening airway disease that might lead to debilitating sequelae such as bronchiectasis and cor pulmonale.

Feline Asthma/Bronchitis

Pathophysiology

Feline bronchial disease is a disorder associated with airway inflammation that results in excessive mucus production, epithelial hyperplasia, and airway smooth muscle constriction.

Over time, airway remodeling results in a physically smaller airway lumen. The subsequent reduction in airway diameter is responsible for the clinical signs of cough and/or respiratory distress seen in affected cats. Acute respiratory distress is associated with bronchoconstriction of hyperresponsive airways.

Disease prevalence has not been established but inflammatory airway disease is encountered frequently in the cat population and it is the most common cause of cough. Etiologic factors that induce airway inflammation have not been elucidated in the naturally occurring disease; however, sensitization to antigen or allergen results in similar clinical and radiographic features of disease. In a small study, cats with respiratory disease had significantly more serum and intradermal responses to a wide variety of allergens (grass, weed, mold, and trees) than cats lacking observable respiratory tract disease (Moriello et al. 2007); however, allergy testing in the cat is fraught with difficulty and inconsistent results. Other factors that have been suggested to play a role in the initiation or perpetuation of airway inflammation include genetic susceptibility, exposure to environmental pollutants or irritants, oxidant-mediated damage, and gastroesophageal reflux.

History and signalment

All ages of cats are affected, although middle-aged females (2–8 years) seem to be more frequently represented. Siamese may have an increased incidence of disease and may suffer from a more chronic form of bronchial disease. Coughing and/or respiratory distress are the most frequently encountered complaints in cats with bronchial disease, and the duration of illness, severity of signs, and presence of other clinical abnormalities are variable. The cough is often described as a dry, "hacking" cough, and paroxysms of coughing with marked abdominal effort may be reported. Some cats may be observed to cough just once a day but this low frequency may not correlate with the degree of airway inflammation present. Owners may report audible breathing sounds or wheezes that become progressively worse over time. Exercise intolerance may be evident, and the cat may limit its activity to lessen the stress on the respiratory system. Cats that develop bronchoconstriction usually display acute respiratory distress, tachypnea, and occasionally cyanosis.

Environmental history is important in cats with bronchial disease, and astute owners may be able to identify trigger events that result in bronchoconstriction. Coughing and respiratory difficulty may worsen in association with use of aerosol sprays, the presence of cigarette smoke, or increased dust in the environment. Avoidance of these triggers can lessen bronchoconstrictive episodes and reduce cough.

Physical examination

Cats with airway disease may appear normal at rest and can have normal pulmonary auscultation. However, these cats will usually display increased tracheal sensitivity, and posttussive crackles can be auscultated. Harsh lung sounds, crackles, or expiratory wheezes can be heard intermittently in affected cats, and the expiratory phase of respiration may be prolonged. Air trapping can occur distal to obstructed airways leading to a barrel-shaped chest. Auscultation in this area of the lung will be relatively quiet, and increased resonance is found on percussion. The remainder of the physical examination is typically normal.

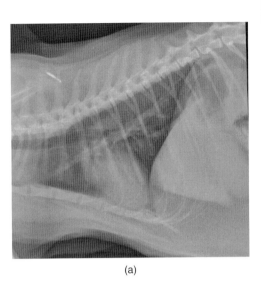

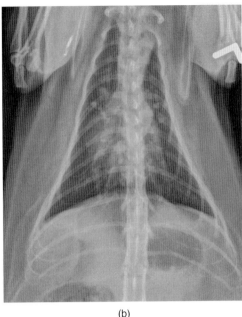

(a)   (b)

Figure 5.16.   Right lateral (a) and dorsoventral (b) radiographs from a 3-year-old FS Abyssinian presented for cough demonstrate a marked, diffuse bronchial pattern. Bronchoalveolar lavage cytology revealed 80% eosinophils.

Diagnostic findings

Cats with bronchial disease or feline asthma may have a neutrophilic leukocytosis. Peripheral eosinophilia is a variable finding. A biochemical profile may reveal hyperproteinemia as a nonspecific indicator of chronic inflammation. Specific tests are required to rule out parasitic bronchitis with *Aelurostrongylus* (see parasitic bronchitis), feline heartworm disease (see Chapter 8), and infectious bronchitis (*Mycoplasma* or *Bordetella*).

The classic radiographic finding in feline bronchial disease is thickening of airways (Figure 5.16); however, radiographs can appear relatively normal, may not fit the severity of the clinical presentation, or can appear similar to those found with infectious causes of cough (Foster et al. 2004). Cats with acute bronchoconstriction may lack pulmonary infiltrates but show other radiographic signs of airway obstruction including flattening of the diaphragm, air trapping or hyperlucency. An alveolar pattern (patchy or lobar involving the right middle lung lobe or other lung lobes) may be observed when a mucus plug obstructs a large airway and causes atelectasis (Figure 5.17).

Airway sampling through transoral tracheal wash or bronchoscopy can be used to collect specimens from feline airways and rule out an infectious cause of cough through culture and cytology (see Chapter 2). Pretreatment with terbutaline (orally or subcutaneously) for 6–12 hours prior to airway sampling can improve the safety of the procedure, perhaps by lessening the bronchoconstrictive response to lavage. An eosinophilic tracheal wash specimen is supportive of the diagnosis of feline bronchial disease in a cat with cough; however, nondegenerate neutrophils predominate in many cases of feline bronchial disease and mixed inflammation is also common (Figure 5.18).

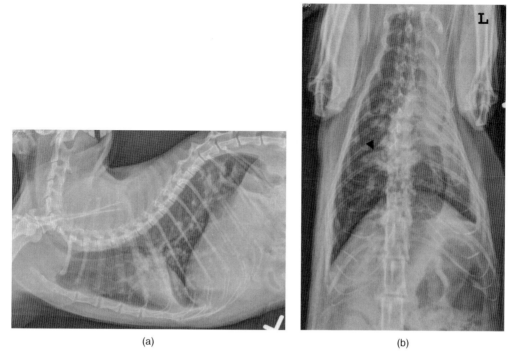

(a)   (b)

Figure 5.17. Left lateral (a) and ventrodorsal (b) radiographs from a 9-year-old MC Siamese with a long-term history of cough. On the lateral view, a lobar sign in the right middle lobe is noted along with diffuse bronchial infiltrates. The ventrodorsal view reveals collapse of the right middle lung lobe (arrowhead) as well as collapse of the left cranial lung lobe (cranial and caudal segments).

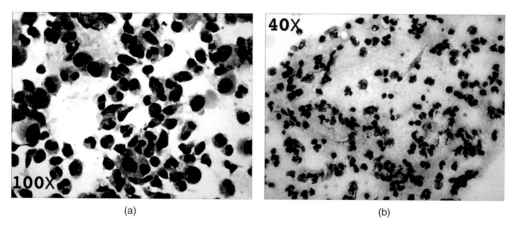

(a)   (b)

Figure 5.18. Bronchoalveolar lavage cytology from two cats with feline bronchial disease reveals primarily eosinophilic inflammation (a) and neutrophilic inflammation in a mucus background (b).

Bacterial cultures should be submitted to rule out infection, although low numbers of bacteria can be isolated from the airways of both healthy and diseased cats because the airways are not always sterile. It is important to rule out *Mycoplasma* infection, which may be a prominent cause of lower respiratory tract infection in cats (Foster et al. 2004).

If airway eosinophilia is documented and owners are interested, consideration could be given to performing allergy testing prior to instituting steroid therapy. Consultation with a local dermatologist is highly recommended because of the difficulty in interpreting results.

Treatment

In the animal that presents with cyanosis and open-mouth breathing, diagnostic tests should be kept to a minimum initially. An oxygen-enriched environment should be provided. Terbutaline, a beta-2-agonist, is an effective bronchodilator and has minimal cardiac side effects. It can be administered subcutaneously or intravenously (0.01 mg/kg) and quickly relieves bronchoconstriction by functionally opposing smooth muscle contraction. Respiratory rate and effort should be monitored visually during the first 15–30 minutes after treatment to determine the therapeutic response. If the cat fails to improve, a second dose of terbutaline can be administered. Short-acting steroids should be administered if the cat remains in respiratory distress and bronchial disease remains highest on the differential list. Steroid therapy is not recommended initially because it will reduce ingress of eosinophils into the airway, thus changing the cytology of subsequent tracheal wash or bronchoalveolar lavage. If the cat fails to respond to bronchodilators and steroids, an alternate etiology of respiratory distress is likely.

Anti-inflammatory agents

Chronic management of feline bronchial disease relies on the judicious use of steroids to control inflammation. The duration and dose of corticosteroid therapy are adjusted according to the severity of respiratory distress in the patient and the rapidity of response to treatment. Initially, prednisolone is administered orally at ~1 mg/kg BID for 5–14 days. The dosage may be decreased to 0.5 mg/kg BID or 1.0 mg/kg daily for 10–20 days if clinical signs are adequately reduced in severity. The dosage can be further tapered over time but most cats appear to require lifelong medication. Recurrent episodes of coughing or respiratory distress necessitate a return to the higher dosage of steroid that controlled clinical signs. Repeat diagnostic testing may also be indicated to ensure the proper diagnosis. Cats are relatively resistant to the side effects of corticosteroids; however, diabetes or congestive heart failure can result from treatment, and an attempt should be made to achieve the lowest dose of the drug that will control signs. Long-acting steroids offer no benefit in control of signs of bronchial disease and tend to result in poor long-term control of inflammation.

Inhaled steroids are also effective in treatment of lower airway inflammatory disease (see Chapter 3). In cats with moderate-to-severe clinical manifestations of disease, oral steroids are recommended during the first 2 weeks of inhaled therapy for more rapid control of disease.

Bronchodilators

Cats that develop acute bronchoconstriction may require periodic treatment with a bronchodilator to alleviate smooth muscle constriction. Selective beta-2-agonists such as terbutaline would be preferred and this drug is easily administered subcutaneously in an emergency situation or at home. Albuterol inhalers are also available for use with the pediatric spacer and facemask, although regular use of specific forms of albuterol could potentially worsen airway inflammation (see Chapter 3). Beta-agonists are not recommended as sole treatment for cats with asthma or bronchitis.

Sustained release theophylline (~15–20 mg/kg orally once daily in the evening) can also be used in the cat. Although it has weak bronchodilatory properties, it may reduce the dose of steroid required to control signs or have other beneficial effects on the respiratory tract (see Chapter 3).

Adjunct therapy

Weight loss should be encouraged in obese cats. Similar to treatment of dogs with chronic bronchitis, saline nebulization, and use of mucolytic agents to encourage evacuation of mucus from the lower airways can be beneficial. Therapies used in humans such as leukotriene agents are not indicated for treatment of cats with bronchial disease. Allergen-specific rush immunotherapy has proven successful in resolution of airway eosinophilia in cats with experimentally induced allergic asthma (Lee-Fowler et al. 2009), however clinical application has not been reported.

Prognosis

Feline bronchial disease is associated with substantial morbidity and even mortality in the feline population. Many cats are well controlled with medication; however, it must be given lifelong in most cats. Cats that experience bronchoconstrictive attacks appear to be most likely to die from the disease or from euthanasia due to the cost of repeated veterinary visits.

Neoplastic Disorders

Pathophysiology

Multiple tumor types can affect the larynx and airways and include lymphosarcoma, squamous cell carcinoma, adenocarcinoma, plasmacytoma, melanoma, chondrosarcoma, and osteochondroma (a benign neoplasm).

History and signalment

Lymphoma and osteochrondroma tend to affect younger animals, and other tumors are typically found in middle-aged to older animals. Malignant tumors of the airways can result in systemic signs of lethargy, anorexia, and weight loss or may cause clinical complaints associated with airway obstruction including dysphonia, dysphagia, and loud or difficult breathing. Cough or collapse associated with airway obstruction can also be reported.

Physical examination

Obstruction of airways dominates the clinical picture. When a large airway is affected, inspiratory prolongation and auscultation of loud inspiratory sounds over the larger airways would be expected. A large mass in a large or central airway can also result in expiratory obstruction and expiratory sounds. Stridor might be detected over the larynx or trachea on inspiration and/or expiration. Obstruction of more distal airways can result in variable auscultatory findings and an abnormal respiratory pattern may or may not be present.

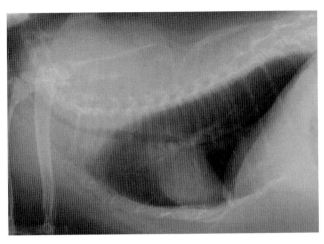

Figure 5.19. Right lateral radiograph from a 10–year-old FS DSH presented for inspiratory and expiratory difficulty. A mass is evident in the tracheal lumen at the fourth rib.

Diagnostic findings

Cervical and thoracic radiography may reveal a mass lesion obstructing the air column in the cervical or intrathoracic region (Figure 5.19). In the laryngeal area, it can be difficult to differentiate a mass lesion from other structures, and ultrasonography should be considered to investigate the region and to obtain an aspirate if possible. In most cases, laryngoscopy or bronchoscopy will be required to define a mass lesion and obtain a biopsy sample for diagnosis (Figure 5.20). If a laryngeal or cervical tracheal mass is suspected, a temporary tracheostomy may be required to secure the airway during analysis of the sample and recovery from anesthesia. For lower airway masses, an oxygen delivery catheter can be passed below the lesion while preparations are made for surgical resection and anastomosis where possible. Obtaining a computed tomography prior to intervention can be helpful in defining the site and extent of the lesion.

If lymphoma is diagnosed, full staging should be performed with abdominal ultrasound and bone marrow aspiration.

Treatment

Debulking of an obstructive lesion can provide some palliation of signs. Lymphosarcoma is treated with radiation and/or chemotherapy, and the availability of chemotherapy for other types of neoplasms depends on the cell of origin. When possible, isolated masses should be surgically resected with wide margins.

Prognosis

Prognosis depends on the tumor type and treatment available. Surgical resection can be curative if metastases are not present, and lymphoma in the airways responds to chemotherapy as it does at other anatomic sites. However, many affected animals are euthanized because of severe airway obstruction that cannot be managed.

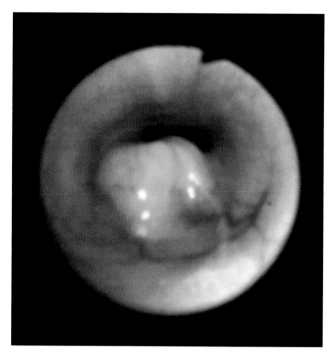

Figure 5.20. Bronchoscopic image from the cat in Figure 5.19 shows a fleshy, lobulated mass filling ~85% of the tracheal lumen.

References

Bauer NB, Schneider MA, Neiger R, Moritz A. Liver disease in dogs with tracheal collapse. J Vet Int Med. 2006; 20(4): 845–849.

Braund KG, Shores A, Cochrane S, Forrester D, Kwiecien JM, Steiss JE. Laryngeal paralysis–polyneuropathy complex in young Dalmatians. Am J Vet Res. 1994; 55(4): 534–542.

Buback JL, Boothe HW, Hobson HP. Surgical treatment of tracheal collapse in dogs: 90 cases (1983–1993). J Am Vet Med Assoc. 1996; 208: 380–384.

Crawford PC, Dubovi EJ, Castleman WL, et al. Transmission of equine influenza virus to dogs. Science. 2005; 310(5747): 482–485.

Foster SF, Martin P, Allan GS, et al. Lower respiratory tract infections in cats: 21 cases (1995–2000). J Feline Med Surg. 2004; 6(3): 167–180.

Gabriel A, Poncelet L, Van Ham L, et al. Laryngeal paralysis–polyneuropathy complex in young related Pyrenean mountain dogs. J Small Anim Pract. 2006; 47(3): 144–149.

Jeffrey ND, Talbot E, Smith PM, et al. Acquired idiopathic laryngeal paralysis as a prominent feature of generalized neuromuscular disease in 39 dogs. Vet Record. 2006; 158: 17–21.

Ledbetter EC, Dubovi EJ, Kim SG, et al. Experimental primary ocular canine herpesvirus-1 infection in adult dogs. Am J Vet Res. 2009; 70(4): 513–512.

Lee-Fowler TM, Cohn LA, DeClue AE, et al. Evaluation of subcutaneous versus mucosal (intranasal) allergen-specific rush immunotherapy in experimental feline asthma. Vet Immunol Immunopathol. 2009; 129(1–2): 49–56.

MacPhail CM, Monnet E. Outcome of and postoperative complications in dogs undergoing surgical treatment of laryngeal paralysis: 140 cases (1985–1998). J Am Vet Med Assoc. 2001; 218(12): 1949–1956.

Macready DM, Johnson LR, Pollard RE. Fluoroscopic and radiographic evaluation of tracheal collapse in dogs: 62 cases (2001–2006). J Am Vet Med Assoc. 2007 15; 230(12): 1870–1876.

Mahony OM, Knowles KE, Braund KG, Averill DR, Jr, Frimberger AE. Laryngeal paralysis-polyneuropathy complex in young Rottweilers. J Vet Intern Med. 1998; 12(5): 330–337.

Mantis P, Lamb CR, Boswood A. Assessment of the accuracy of thoracic radiography in the diagnosis of canine chronic bronchitis. J Small Anim Pract. 1998; 39: 518–520.

Moriello KA, Stepien RL, Henik RA, Wenholz LJ. Pilot study: prevalence of positive aeroallergen reactions in 10 cats with small-airway disease without concurrent skin disease. Vet Dermatol. 2007; 18(2): 94–100.

Moritz A, Schneider M, Bauer N. Management of advanced tracheal collapse in dogs using intraluminal self-expanding biliary wallstents. J Vet Int Med. 2004; 18(1): 31–42.

O'Brien JA, Hendricks J. Inherited laryngea paralysis: analysis in the Husky cross. Vet Q 1986; 8: 301–302.

Peeters DE, McKiernan BC, Weisiger RM, et al. Quantitative bacterial cultures and cytological examination of bronchoalveolar lavage specimens in dogs. J Vet Int Med. 2000; 14: 534–541.

Ridyard AE, Corcoran BM, Tasker S, et al. Spontaneous laryngeal paralysis in four white-coated German shepherd dogs. J Small Anim Pract. 2000; 41(12): 558–561.

Shelton GD, Podell M, Poncelet L, et al. Inherited polyneuropathy in Leonberger dogs: A mixed or intermediate form of Charcot-Marie-Tooth disease? Muscle Nerve. 2003; 27(4): 471–477.

Sura PA, Krahwinkel DJ. Self-expanding nitinol stents for the treatment of tracheal collapse in dogs: 12 cases (2001–2004). J Am Vet Med Assoc. 2008 15; 232(2): 228–236.

Tasker S, Foster DJ, Corcoran BM, et al. Obstructive inflammatory laryngeal disease in three cats. J Feline Med Surg. 1999 1(1): 53–59.

Venker van-Haagen AJ, Hartman W, Goedegebuure SA. Spontaneous laryngeal paralysis in young Bouviers. J Am Anim Hosp Assoc. 1978; 14: 714–720.

Weisse CWC. Intraluminal stenting for tracheal collapse. In Current Veterinary Therapy XIV, Bonagura J, Twedt D (eds). Saunders Elsevier, New York. 2009, pp 635–641.

Parenchymal Disease

6

Structural Diseases

Primary Ciliary Dyskinesia

Pathophysiology

Normal cilia are made up of nine pairs of microtubules surrounding a central pair. Inner and outer dynein arms connect the microtubules, and the enzyme dynein splits ATP to provide energy for ciliary motility. Primary ciliary dyskinesia (PCD) is a congenital or inherited disorder that is most often associated with a defect in the dynein arms (total or partial absence) resulting in defective ciliary motion. All organs that contain cilia are affected including the respiratory tract, middle ear, and reproductive tract. PCD that is accompanied by *situs inversus* and bronchiectasis is referred to as Kartagener's syndrome.

History and signalment

PCD has been reported in related Bichon Frise, English pointers, Springer Spaniels, Newfoundland, Old English Sheepdogs, and other breeds. It is rarely reported in the cat. Clinical signs can be seen in puppies as early as 5 weeks of age, or animals may be older when the severity or recurrence of signs triggers evaluation. Historical complaints include chronic or recurrent sneezing, serous to mucoid nasal discharge, chronic cough, and episodes of antibiotic-responsive pneumonia. Signs of otitis media (head tilt, aural discharge, or nystagmus) or infertility may also be reported.

Physical examination

Bilateral serous to mucopurulent nasal discharge is common and dogs may display evidence of pneumonia with a moist cough on tracheal palpation, increased tracheal sensitivity, and increased bronchovesicular sounds. Severely affected animals can be cyanotic. Nonrespiratory abnormalities that may be found include hydrocephalus and otitis media.

Diagnosis

A complete blood count may be supportive of bronchopneumonia, with alterations in neutrophil numbers, and thoracic radiographs reveal alveolar infiltrates during bouts of pneumonia. Airway sampling typically reveals a septic suppurative response and infection with *Mycoplasma* and aerobic bacteria (*Pasteurella, Streptococcus,* and *Staphylococcus)* is common. Diagnosis of PCD requires documentation of functional and structural defects of cilia. In an intact male dog with the appropriate clinical history, lack of purposeful sperm motility is consistent with a diagnosis of PCD. Respiratory ciliary function is assessed through tracheal scintigraphy using 99-technetium-labeled macroaggregated albumin deposited at the carina. Ciliary movement of the radiolabel is followed with a gamma camera, and animals with ciliary dyskinesia have no motion detected. *Mycoplasma* and *Bordetella* infections should be appropriately treated prior to performing tracheal scintigraphy because infection with these organisms causes ciliostasis and could result in a false-positive scintigraphic study.

Nasal or tracheal biopsies or a semen sample fixed in glutaraldehyde can be submitted for electron microscopy to identify the characteristic ultrastructural abnormalities seen in PCD; however, electron microscopy is not widely available and a properly sectioned sample is critical to assess ciliary structures. A pathologist should be consulted prior to obtaining a biopsy to insure that an adequate sample is obtained and that a proper interpretation can be provided. Dogs with PCD will have multiple defects in cilia (loss or shortening of dynein arms, loss of central pair of microtubules, triplets in place of doublets, etc.) and will have >5–20% of cilia affected. Findings must be distinguished from those of acquired or secondary ciliary abnormalities, which can be found with a variety of chronic respiratory tract diseases. These secondary defects typically affect <5% of the affected cilia, and compound cilia (multiple cilia contained within a single membranous layer) are often prominent. In human patients, PCD can occur in the absence of specific electron microscopy abnormalities and it is likely that this occurs in veterinary patients also, although it has not been specifically documented.

Treatment

Aggressive therapy for pneumonia is required and owners should be taught to recognize recurrence of disease so that treatment can be instituted immediately. Intermittent or sustained respiratory therapy with nebulization and coupage can be used to encourage clearance of respiratory secretions. Cough suppressants should not be used because of the risk for trapping infected secretions in the lower airways and promoting the development of secondary bronchiectasis.

Prognosis

Many dogs with PCD are able to survive multiple bouts of pneumonia and develop fewer episodes as they mature; however, they remain at risk for recurrent infection. If pneumonia is insufficiently treated, bronchiectasis may develop. Contact with other animals that might serve as a source of infection should be limited. Affected dogs should not be used in the breeding pool and genetic counseling is recommended.

Lung Lobe Torsion

Pathophysiology

The precise etiology of lung lobe torsion is unknown. It may be associated with atelectasis of a lobe from bronchial obstruction (by mucus impaction or a neoplasm) and twisting of the lobar bronchus on its axis. Lobar consolidation due to infection might also predispose to torsion. Alternately, it is possible that pleural effusion precedes lung lobe torsion, causing collapse of a lung lobe and an environment that allows the lobe to twist along the bronchial axis.

Typically, venous compression caused by the torsion leads to congestion and swelling of the lung lobe. This could then cause pleural effusion, which is commonly, but not always, found with lung lobe torsion. Pleural effusion is often hemorrhagic or chylous in character. The lobes most commonly affected by torsion are the right middle lung lobe (particularly in large-breed dogs) and the left cranial lung lobe (in Pugs and other small-breed dogs).

History and signalment

There is an increased incidence of lung lobe torsion in the Afghan hound and deep-chested dog breeds, although it is also seen in small-breed dogs, with Pugs affected most commonly. Torsion appears to be uncommon in the cat but it has been reported in a cat with chronic, poorly treated lower airway inflammatory disease and was likely preceded by lobar collapse associated with mucus obstruction. Clinical complaints reported with lung lobe torsion include tachypnea or difficulty breathing, lethargy, anorexia, and coughing. In chronic cases, weight loss may be noted.

Physical examination

Tachypnea is a common finding, and Heart and lung sounds can be muffled or absent focally in the region of the torsion or ventrally in the thorax due to the presence of pleural effusion. Elevated body temperature occurs in 50–60% of cases.

Diagnostic findings

Affected animals usually display a neutrophilic leukocytosis due to stress, inflammation, necrosis, or infection. Radiographs reveal pleural effusion in over 80% of cases, and thoracocentesis is indicated to alleviate respiratory distress and improve visualization of thoracic contents. Lobar opacity is a common radiographic finding (Figure 6.1), and an abnormal bronchial position can be visualized in 10–50% of dogs. Thoracic ultrasound with evaluation of pulmonary blood flow may be helpful in some cases although the most common finding appears to be hepatization of the lung lobe. A vesicular gas pattern is seen on

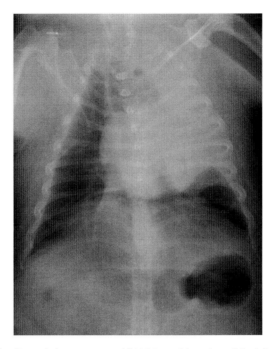

Figure 6.1. Dorsoventral radiograph from a 3-year-old MC Pug with torsion of the left cranial lung lobe. Note the absence of pleural effusion in this case.

radiographs, ultrasound, or computed tomography. Bronchoscopy can document lung lobe torsion as the cause for lobar consolidation through visualization a twisted appearance to the bronchial opening.

Thoracic fluid analysis reveals chyle (see Chapter 7) in up to one-third of dogs and a modified transudate, hemorrhage, or exudate has been reported in the remaining cases (Neath et al. 2000). Cytology of the fluid is indicated to rule out infectious or neoplastic disease, and samples should be evaluated by aerobic and anaerobic bacterial culture. Histopathology of lung tissue usually shows pulmonary hemorrhage, inflammation, and infarction but may reveal a primary disease process responsible for the torsion such as neoplasia or bronchial obstruction.

Treatment

Lung lobectomy is required for appropriate treatment. The lobe should not be de-rotated prior to removal because of the risk for ischemic injury associated with reperfusion.

Prognosis

Over 50% of dogs will have an uncomplicated recovery from lung lobectomy; however, some dogs will experience persistent chylothorax that necessitates further intervention. Torsion of a second lung lobe can also occur.

Infectious Diseases

Viral Pneumonia

Pathophysiology

Etiologic agents of viral pneumonia in the dog include canine distemper virus (CDV) and canine influenza virus (CIV). Less commonly, canine parainfluenza virus-3 (PI-3), canine adenovirus-2 (CAV-2), canine herpesvirus (CHV-1), and canine respiratory coronavirus (CRCoV) can cause parenchymal infection but these organisms more typically result in airway disease (see Chapter 5). In the cat, feline calicivirus (FCV) is the most common viral cause of pneumonia, although feline herpesvirus-1 (FHV-1) can cause a severe tracheitis and pneumonia.

Viruses are spread by inhalation of aerosolized viral particles that gain access to the lower respiratory tract. These viruses cause diffuse epithelial cell death and provoke an inflammatory response primarily within the interstitium. Most viral infections are self-limiting but predispose animals to bacterial bronchopneumonia and thus can lead to more severe systemic signs.

Noneffusive feline infectious peritonitis (FIP) virus (the mutated coronavirus) can cause a granulomatous pneumonia due to immune mediated vasculitis and pyogranulomatous response rather than due to an infectious process (see Chapter 7).

History and signalment

Puppies and kittens are more susceptible to most viral agents than adult animals with the exception of canine influenza virus, which tends to affect mature dogs. Generally clinical signs are acute in onset and associated primarily with cough. Animals held in close confinement are more prone to infection. CDV results in more severe clinical and systemic signs of illness and is characterized by concurrent or sequential development of gastrointestinal and neurologic signs (typically myoclonus).

Physical examination

Dogs or cats with viral pneumonia may have fever and/or tachypnea that ranges from mild to severe. Lung sounds may be slightly harsh and tracheal sensitivity is usually found. Dogs with CDV may have retinochoroiditis or neurologic deficits that involve the cerebrum, cerebellum, or spinal cord.

Diagnostic findings

Diagnosis is often based on clinical suspicion, history and signalment, environmental exposure, and vaccination status. A CBC may reveal lymphopenia early in viral infection. Viral pneumonia is expected to result in a diffuse interstitial pattern on chest radiographs, although bacterial complications can lead to alveolar infiltrates.

Various methods can be used to confirm the presence of virus or exposure to a virus; however, it can be more difficult to determine if the virus is the cause of the disease (see CIRD, Chapter 5). Airway wash fluid or pulmonary tissue can be analyzed by fluorescent antibody staining or application of immunohistochemistry to fixed tissue can identify virus-specific antigen; however, tests are not widely available for all viruses and can be difficult to perform. Also, electron microscopy can be used to detect viral inclusions.

Treatment

General supportive care measures are instituted including subcutaneous or intravenous fluid therapy, airway humidification, and oxygen therapy as needed. Affected animals are kept segregated from other animals to avoid spread of disease. No specific antiviral therapy is generally recommended; however, broad-spectrum antibiotics are often administered to treat or to prevent secondary bacterial infection. *Mycoplasma* spp. are commonly found in conjunction with suspected viral infection, thus doxycycline or azithromycin would be appropriate for use.

Prognosis

Regular vaccination protects against most of the viral infections that can result in pneumonia. In general, viral pneumonia has a good prognosis as most animals will respond to supportive care and treatment of secondary bacterial pneumonia. Dogs with distemper virus that develop neurologic disease have a poor prognosis in general, although some will survive.

Bacterial Pneumonia

Pathophysiology

Bacterial pneumonia occurs when increased numbers of opportunistic pathogens overwhelm host defense mechanisms or when highly pathogenic organisms gain access to the airways. It can also result from failure of respiratory defense mechanisms, systemic immune compromise, or inhalation of a foreign body or caustic substance. Therefore, in the animal with bacterial pneumonia, a search should begin for an underlying disease or predisposing disorder that allows parenchymal infection. Enteric organisms are the most common bacteria found in lower respiratory tract infections in adult dogs and are implicated (along with *Bordetella*) in community-acquired pneumonia in puppies. Exposure to primary respiratory pathogens (*Bordetella* or *Mycoplasma*) can result in lung infection and life-threatening pneumonia in kittens and puppies.

Bacterial colonization of the respiratory epithelium incites chemotaxis of neutrophils. These inflammatory cells release proteolytic enzymes and reactive oxygen species to kill the bacteria; however, this process sets up an inflammatory environment within the lung. A delicate balance develops between control of bacterial growth and lung inflammation. In some cases, overwhelming inflammation perpetuates lung damage, resulting in gas-exchange abnormalities that can lead to respiratory failure.

History and signalment

Pneumonia is encountered at any age of animal. Puppies are most commonly affected by community-acquired pneumonia, young hunting or sporting dogs are most commonly affected by foreign body pneumonia, and older animals develop pneumonia in association with aspiration injury or immune compromise. Certain dog breeds are predisposed to infectious pneumonia. For example, Irish Wolfhounds develop an unusual rhinitis/bronchopneumonia syndrome (Clercx et al. 2003). The reason that some of these dogs have a propensity for bacterial pneumonia is unclear but may be related to a heritable immunodeficiency.

Dogs or cats with bacterial pneumonia generally have an acute history of a productive cough, labored breathing, and respiratory difficulty or distress. However, some animals present with more chronic and vague signs of illness such as malaise, depression, anorexia, and weight loss. Nasal discharge is sometimes the primary complaint when animals cough respiratory secretions into the nasopharynx or have coincident nasal infection.

Physical examination

Abnormalities indicative of bacterial pneumonia are found in the examination of the respiratory tract. Parenchymal infection with alveolar flooding by inflammatory debris leads to restrictive lung disease, and a rapid shallow breathing pattern typically results. Depending on the stage and severity of disease, thoracic auscultation usually reveals adventitious lung sounds (crackles or wheezes) or loud, harsh bronchovesicular sounds. Absence of lung sounds in a specific region of the thorax might be suggestive of lung consolidation or pleuropneumonia.

A mucopurulent nasal discharge can be present in some animals. Although pneumonia is an inflammatory condition, fever is detected in <50% of affected adult dogs or puppies (Radhakrishnan et al. 2007).

Diagnostic findings

Leukocytosis with a left shift supports the diagnosis of bacterial pneumonia in an animal with appropriate clinical findings. Neutropenia with a degenerative left shift can occur if acute fulminant pneumonia results in pulmonary sequestration of neutrophils. A biochemical profile and urinalysis assist in the diagnosis of underlying conditions such as diabetes mellitus and hyperadrenocorticism, which are associated with defective neutrophil function and might rarely predispose the animal to pneumonia. FeLV/FIV serology should be performed in cats with pneumonia, although a direct association has not been made between viral status and the development of bacterial pneumonia.

Pulse oximetry should be employed to determine the severity of lung dysfunction as well as the need for oxygen supplementation because hypoxemia is common in animals with moderate to severe disease. SPO_2 can also be used to follow response to therapy, although an arterial blood gas provides a more accurate assessment of oxygenation (see Chapter 2).

Thoracic radiographs obtained in the early stages of bacterial pneumonia may demonstrate mild or diffuse interstitial infiltrates. Alveolar infiltrates with air bronchograms are considered the classic radiographic finding (Figure 6.2). In severe cases, these infiltrates can coalesce to cause lobar consolidation. A lobar infiltrate can also be suggestive of foreign body pneumonia. Pleuropneumonia is uncommon in small animals unless a pleural foreign body or bite wound is the cause of pneumonia. In these cases, infection with *Actinomyces* can be found.

Direct airway sampling through tracheal wash, bronchoscopy with bronchoalveolar lavage, or fine-needle aspiration of the lung is indicated to confirm the etiology of pneumonia

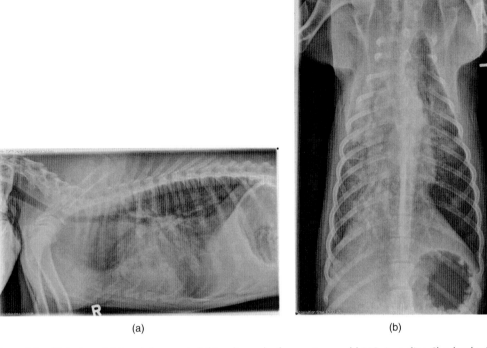

(a)   (b)

Figure 6.2.   Right lateral (a) and dorsoventral (b) radiographs from a 7-year-old MC Australian Shepherd with bronchopneumonia affecting primarily the right lung lobe. Air bronchograms are visible in both views primarily in the right lung lobe. Nodular densities likely represent metastatic lung disease.

and to obtain samples for Gram stain, aerobic and anaerobic bacterial culture with antibiotic sensitivity testing, *Mycoplasma* culture, and cytology. Of these techniques, tracheal wash is most suited for radiographically diffuse disease, while bronchoscopy (Figure 6.3) or fine-needle lung aspiration would be preferred for focal disease (see Chapter 2). Gram staining characteristics and cytology can be useful for identifying the most likely infecting organism and initiating early antibiotic therapy.

Various bacteria can be recovered from airways of healthy cats and dogs, although only cats with pulmonary disease have had *Mycoplasma* isolated from lower airways to date. Therefore, documentation of pneumonia requires isolation of bacteria in conjunction with detection of septic suppurative inflammation on airway cytology (Figure 6.4). Pneumonia in the dog is usually caused by Gram-negative enteric bacteria (Table 6.1). Multiple species are isolated in almost half of all cases, and 22% of infections are complicated by the presence of anaerobic bacteria (Angus et al. 1997). Bacterial pneumonia is clinically recognized much less commonly in the cat than in the dog, and less information is available about potential causes, although it appears that *Bordetella* and *Mycoplasma* spp. are commonly involved in conjunction with *Pasteurella* spp (Bart et al. 2000) (Table 6.2). A more recent study also implicated *Mycoplasma* spp. as the most common isolate in feline pneumonia (Foster et al. 2004).

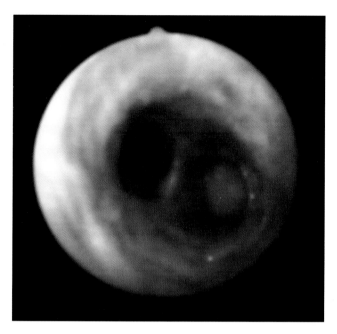

Figure 6.3.   Bronchoscopy image from a dog with *Mycoplasma* pneumonia reveals airway hyperemia and marked mucus plugging of an isolated airway.

Treatment

While waiting to obtain results of cultures, antibiotic treatment should be initiated by using antibiotics likely to be effective against the organisms involved. The combination of a fluoroquinolone and penicillin derivative is used most commonly for initial therapy. Antibiotics

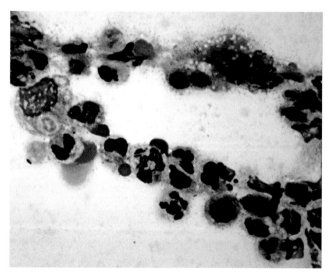

Figure 6.4.   This image of airway cytology confirms bacterial pneumonia by the presence of dark blue rod-shaped bacteria within neutrophils. Note the swollen nuclei and degenerate changes in neutrophils throughout the slide. Bacterial culture identified *E. coli.*

Table 6.1. Bacterial organisms commonly found in dogs with lower respiratory tract infection (Angus 1997)

Isolate	Number of Samples	Gram-Stain characteristics
Enteric group	53 (46%)	Gram-negative rods
Escherichia coli	36 (31%)	
Klebsiella	8 (7%)	
Other enterics	15 (13%)	
Pasteurella species	26 (22%)	Gram-negative rods
β-Hemolytic *Streptococcus*	14 (12%)	Gram-positive cocci
Streptococcus/Enterococcus	14 (12%)	Gram-positive cocci
Obligate anaerobes	25 (22%)	Gram-positive or -negative
Bordetella bronchiseptica	14 (12%)	Gram-negative coccobacilli
Coagulase + *Staphylococcus*	11 (10%)	Gram-positive cocci
Pseudomonas species	9 (8%)	Gram-negative rods
Mycoplasma	6 (5%)	None (no cell wall)
Other	18 (16%)	

are usually required for >3 weeks, and long-term treatment is based on results obtained from culture and susceptibility testing. Clinical signs, pulse oximetry, and radiographic changes are used to determine when therapy can be discontinued.

Bronchodilators are sometimes considered for animals with pneumonia. These drugs can reduce the work of breathing and improve diaphragmatic strength; however, the potential for gastrointestinal toxicity associated with a methylxanthine drug or beta-agonist must be considered. Also, use of enrofloxacin in combination with theophylline can result in higher plasma levels of theophylline and potential toxicity.

Generalized supportive care and ancillary respiratory therapy will aid in resolution of pneumonia. Oxygen supplementation is beneficial in decreasing respiratory effort and improving clinical status. Promoting systemic hydration through use of intravenous fluids is very important for maintaining hydration of respiratory secretions and facilitating their removal from the respiratory tree. Saline nebulization followed by coupage is also beneficial

Table 6.2. Bacterial organisms commonly found in cats with lower respiratory tract infection (Bart et al. 2000)

Isolate	Number of Samples	Gram-Stain Characteristics
Bordetella bronchiseptica	12 (30%)	Gram-negative coccobacilli
Pasteurella species	9 (22%)	Gram-negative rods
Mycoplasma	6 (15%)	None (no cell wall)
Escherichia coli	5 (12%)	Gram-negative rods
Streptococcus	6 (15%)	Gram-positive cocci
Other	2 (5%)	
Obligate anaerobes	1 (unknown percentage)	

in treatment of pneumonia by providing direct hydration of the lower airways. See Chapter 3 for more information.

Prognosis

In an animal with nonresolving pneumonia, the possibility of a foreign body, pulmonary abscess, or underlying neoplastic process should be considered. In these cases, lung lobectomy is a viable option for management of disease, although some dogs can have persistence of disease despite surgery. In one study, over half of the animals treated with lung lobectomy had resolution of disease (Murphy et al. 1997).

Fungal Pneumonia

Pathophysiology

Organisms most commonly involved in systemic mycotic infections are thermally dimorphic fungi, existing as molds in the environment with transformation into yeasts following inhalation into the respiratory tract. The fungal organisms involved are characterized by specific geographic distribution. *Histoplasma capsulatum* and *Blastomyces dermatitidis* are found primarily in the Ohio/Mississippi river valley. *Coccidioides immitis* is found in the southwestern United States. Other fungal organisms that occasionally cause pneumonia include *Cryptococcus*, *Aspergillus*, and *Conidiobolus*. *Pneumocystis* is a rare cause of fungal pneumonia and is discussed under protozoal and other pneumonias because the clinical syndrome is different from that of other mycotic infections.

Fungal organisms differ in geographic distribution and also in tissue trophism. In addition to pulmonary infection, all organisms tend to affect peripheral and internal lymph nodes; ocular and central nervous tissue may also be involved. *Histoplasma* also infects the gastrointestinal tract, liver, spleen, and bone marrow, while *Blastomyces* has a predilection for bone, skin, and the reproductive tract. *C. immitis* infects bone and cardiac structures. In cats, *Coccidioides* and *Histoplasma* frequently cause skin lesions (Greene and Troy 1995).

History and signalment

Dogs are infected with fungal pneumonia more frequently than cats and most animals are young, outdoor-hunting breeds. A variety of historical complaints can be reported depending on the organ(s) affected and include cough, tachypnea, respiratory distress, weight loss, diarrhea, blindness, glaucoma, lameness, skin lesions, and neurologic signs.

Physical examination

Abnormalities detected in the respiratory tract include labored respirations, tachypnea, and harsh crackles or loud bronchial noises. Wheezing can be present when hilar lymphadenopathy results in bronchial compression. Tracheal sensitivity is usually present. Ocular lesions include glaucoma, anterior uveitis, and chorioretinitis. Both central and peripheral neurologic deficits can be noted. Ulcerated, draining skin lesions, peripheral lymphadenopathy, testicular or prostatic enlargement, and bone pain can also be found depending on the infecting organism. Histoplasmosis affecting the bone marrow can result in severe

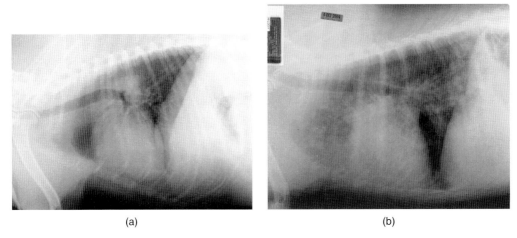

(a)   (b)

Figure 6.5. Lateral radiographs from a dog with coccidioidomycosis (a) and blastomycosis (b). Hilar lymphadenopathy is prominent and a mild interstitial pattern is present throughout (a). A diffuse nodular interstitial pattern is seen characterized by similarly sized nodules throughout the lung lobes (b). (Courtesy of Dr. Melissa Herrera, University of California, Davis.)

thrombocytopenia and petechiation. Hepatosplenomegaly or a thickened gastrointestinal tract can also be found in animals with histoplasmosis.

Diagnostic findings

Fungal infection should be suspected in an animal with multisystemic disease that has a history of travel to an area endemic for a fungal organism. Laboratory testing commonly reveals a mild nonregenerative anemia, neutrophilic and monocytic leukocytosis, hypoalbuminemia associated with chronic disease or gastrointestinal fungal infection, thrombocytopenia due to bone marrow involvement, and potentially hypercalcemia (primarily with blastomycosis).

Chest radiographs reveal hilar lymphadenopathy in the majority of fungal infections. A variety of pulmonary infiltrative patterns are found concurrently including a miliary or nodular infiltrate, generalized interstitial or bronchial pattern, lobar consolidation, or a mass lesion (Figure 6.5).

Serologic assays for most fungal infections (histoplasmosis, blastomycosis, and coccidioidomycosis) are variably useful because animals in endemic regions will usually develop a positive antibody titer due to exposure (Shubitz et al. 2005). However, in a dog or cat with appropriate clinical findings and travel to an area endemic for *C. immitis*, a positive coccidioidomycosis titer can be considered relatively diagnostic, particularly if a quantitative agar gel immunodiffusion test for IgM and IgG (UC Davis) is performed. A recently developed enzyme immunoassay (MiraVista Diagnostics, Indianapolis, IN) using *Blastomyces* galactomannan antigen displayed better sensitivity for confirming disease and can be performed on serum or urine (Spector et al. 2008). Specificity has not yet been assessed and it is possible that this test will cross-react with *Histoplasma* and *Coccidioides*. However, this test may also be useful in monitoring response to therapy because antigen levels were noted to decline with itraconazole treatment.

Table 6.3. Characteristics of common fungal organisms

Fungus	Ecologic Niche	Cytologic Characteristics
Blastomyces dermatidis	Mississippi/Missouri River Valleys	Broad based budding yeast, 5–20 µm, generally extracellular
Histoplasma capsulatum	Mississippi/Missouri River Valleys	2–4 µm, usually found in clusters within macrophages
Coccidioides immitis	Arizona/New Mexico	10–80 µm, double-walled structure containing endospores

Diagnosis of a fungal infection can be made by cytologic or histologic assessment of lymph node or organ aspirates, airway samples obtained by tracheal wash or bronchoalveolar lavage, skin impression smears, aqueous centesis, or bone marrow evaluation. Fungi are of distinctive sizes and shapes and are usually surrounded by pyogranulomatous inflammation (Table 6.3).

Treatment

Depending on the severity and extent of illness, fungistatic or fungicidal therapy might be preferred in an animal with fungal pneumonia (see Chapter 3). Long-term therapy and monitoring are generally required for treatment of fungal infection.

Prognosis

Survival rates for animals with fungal pneumonia are not specifically known, and outcome depends not only on the severity of lung disease but also on the presence of other organ involvement. In addition, surgery is often required for a dog with a painful glaucomatous eye, an intact male dog that might sequester organisms in the prostrate, or a dog with a consolidated lung lobe. Dogs that survive the first week of treatment will most likely be cured of disease. However, approximately 20% of dogs with blastomycosis developed recurrence of disease 4–12 months after a 60-day course of itraconazole (Legendre et al. 1996).

Protozoal and Similar Pneumonias

Pathophysiology

Although rare, pneumonia can result from infection with protozoan organisms such as *Neospora caninum* and *Toxoplasma gondii*. In addition, *Pneumocystis jiroveci*, an organism that shares some characteristics of protozoans but has been classified as a fungal organism, can result in a similar type of pneumonia. *Pneumocystis* are reportedly found in the lungs of normal, healthy individuals and development of infection is typically associated with immunosuppression. In dogs, a combined congenital immunodeficiency is suspected in the Miniature Dachshund (Lobetti 2000) and an immunoglobulin (IgG) deficiency has been proposed in Cavalier King Charles Spaniels (Watson et al. 2006). These organisms lead to pyogranulomatous inflammation and interstitial pneumonia.

History and signalment

Pneumonia due to *Neospora* can be seen in congenitally infected puppies in conjunction with ascending paralysis of the limbs. Disease is associated with a high fatality rate. *Toxoplasma* pneumonia of cats or kittens is usually associated with severe systemic disease and rapidly progresses to death. In the dog, toxoplasmosis is less common but infection can also result in pneumonia. Pneumocystosis has been reported most commonly in Miniature Dachsunds less than 1 year of age and in adult Cavalier King Charles Spaniels, as well as sporadic other breeds. Typical presenting complaints with *Pneumocystis* pneumonia include a chronic cough, progressively worsening exercise intolerance and tachypnea, and gradual weight loss.

Physical examination

Tachypnea with labored or respiration or increased respiratory effort is common. Fever is generally absent or body temperature only mildly elevated, and animals display a poor body condition score. Respiratory auscultation is generally unremarkable and a dry cough can be triggered by tracheal palpation. Systemic or neurologic signs may be seen in animals with toxoplasmosis or neosporosis.

Diagnostic findings

Standard laboratory tests reveal nonspecific findings of neutrophilic leukocytosis. Positive serology for *Neospora* in conjunction with clinical signs provides a presumptive diagnosis. A diagnosis of *Toxoplasma* would be suspected in an animal with relevant clinical findings that has a positive IgM titer or a fourfold increase in IgG titer in conjunction with positive response to treatment. It is rare to document *Toxoplasma* oocysts in the feces. In Cavalier King Charles Spaniels suspected of pneumocystosis, measurement of serum immunoglobulins should be considered.

Thoracic radiographs in protozoal or *Pneumocystis* pneumonia most commonly reveal diffuse interstitial or nodular infiltrates (Figure 6.6), although alveolar densities are occasionally seen. Organisms may be identified in tracheal wash, bronchoalveolar lavage fluid, fine-needle aspirate, or lung biopsy in conjunction with neutrophilic inflammation, although detection of *Neospora* is particularly rare. *Toxoplasma* tachyzoites that may be found in bronchoalveolar lavage fluid are 2×6 µm in length and are found extracellularly or intracellularly within macrophages. *Pneumocystis* organisms appear as trophozoites ranging in size from 1–4 µm or as cysts, which are 5–8 µm in size and contain two to eight small inclusions. Necropsy findings are typically diagnostic.

Treatment

Toxoplasma is most commonly treated with clindamycin (12.5 mg/kg PO BID) or trimethoprim-sulfa (15 mg/kg PO daily to BID) for >4 weeks. Clindamycin might also be effective for *Neospora*. Treatment of *Pneumocystis* pneumonia relies on the use of trimethoprim-sulfamethoxazole at 15–30 mg/kg PO BID–TID for 4 weeks or longer as needed. Dogs treated with trimethoprim-sulfa should be monitored for development of

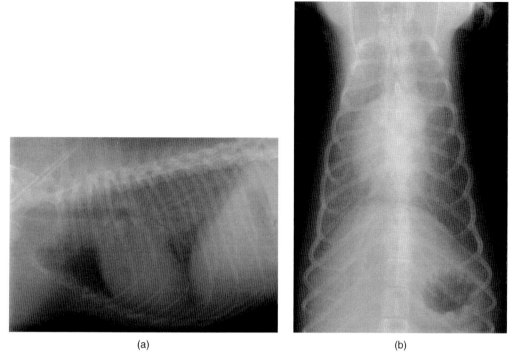

(a)   (b)

Figure 6.6. Right lateral (a) and dorsoventral (b) radiographs from a 2-year-old MC Cavalier King Charles Spaniel with pneumocystosis.

keratoconjunctivitis sicca or anemia due to folate deficiency throughout treatment. Standard supportive care for pneumonia with oxygen supplementation should also be employed as needed.

Prognosis

Pulmonary toxoplasmosis or neosporosis is often fatal in young animals. Young adult Cavaliers with pneumocystosis might have a relatively good prognosis, with survival reported in seven of nine cases (Watson et al. 2006), although other scattered reports suggest <50% survival. It is likely that the degree of lung involvement determines response to therapy (Figure 6.7).

Inflammatory Disorders

Eosinophilic Bronchopneumopathy

Pathophysiology

Eosinophilic lung disease in the dog (EBP: eosinophilic bronchopneumopathy or PIE: pulmonary infiltrates with eosinophilia) is a poorly understood disorder. Heartworm disease, lung parasitism, and larval migration of parasites are recognized causes of eosinophilic

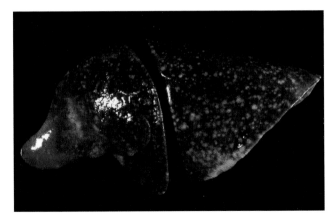

Figure 6.7. Gross necropsy findings from the dog depicted in Figure 6.6 revealed consolidation with hemorrhage throughout the lungs. Small pinpoint to miliary, firm, nodular white foci are evenly distributed throughout all lung lobes. Pyogranulomatous pneumonia with *Pneumocystis* organisms was confirmed histologically.

airway disease; however, primary eosinophilic infiltration of the lung can occur in the absence of an inciting cause. The finding of increased CD[4+] T-cells in BAL fluid suggests that a type 2 hypersensitivity response might be responsible for the idiopathic disease (Clercx et al. 2002), although cytokine profiles in airway tissues from dogs with EBP did not support a Th2 hypersensitivity or allergic response (Peeters et al. 2006).

History and signalment

Dogs with EBP are usually young adults, ranging from ~1 year to 8 years of age and can be of any breed or size, although it seems to occur more commonly in larger breed dogs. In one study, Siberian husky dogs were overrepresented (Clercx et al. 2000). Owner complaints can be present for months to years prior to presentation and generally include a harsh unrelenting cough and progressive respiratory difficulty with exercise intolerance. Some dogs have concurrent nasal discharge or are systemically ill with lethargy and anorexia. Lack of response to antibiotics is common.

Physical examination

Increased lung sounds or harsh crackles and expiratory wheezes can be auscultated in approximately 50% of cases, and tracheal palpation results in a moist productive cough. Some dogs display yellow-green nasal discharge or may expectorate this type of material. Nasal airflow is preserved, regional lymph nodes are normal, and no other physical examination findings are anticipated, although body temperature is sometimes elevated.

Diagnostic findings

Leukocytosis is found in approximately 50% of cases, and peripheral neutrophilia or eosinophilia can be observed. Importantly, while peripheral eosinophilia can be profound in dogs with EBP some will show normal eosinophil counts. When EBP is suspected based on clinical presentation and blood work, parasitism should be ruled out by performing

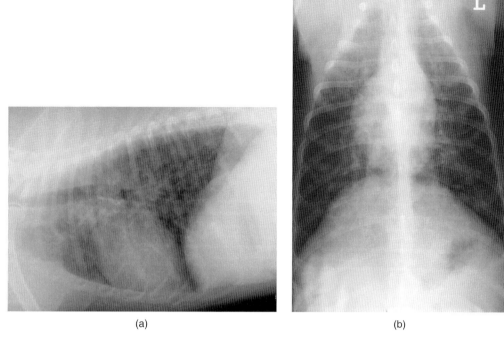

(a)   (b)

Figure 6.8. Right lateral (a) and dorsoventral (b) radiographs from a 2-year-old FS mixed-breed dog with eosinophilic lung disease reveal a severe diffuse bronchial pattern.

heartworm tests and fecal analyses (see parasitic bronchitis, Chapter 5). Pulse oximetry and arterial blood gas analysis (where available) are recommended because hypoxemia can be marked in affected dogs and may persist after clinical and radiographic resolution of disease, suggesting that EBP can be associated with permanent lung damage.

Radiographs in dogs with EBP are generally abnormal, with bronchointerstitial patterns reported most commonly (Figure 6.8). Alveolar infiltrates and bronchiectasis are also encountered frequently. Airway examination is remarkable for yellow-green tinged mucus in some affected dogs, indicating the presence of eosinophils. Mucosal irregularities and airway collapse have also been reported. Other cases may show pronounced airway hyperemia (Figure 6.9). Normal dogs have ~5% eosinophils on a differential count of bronchoalveolar lavage fluid while dogs with EBP can have up to 90% eosinophils (Figure 6.10). Bacterial culture of airway fluid is negative or reveals a light growth of normal flora.

Rhinoscopy has been performed in some dogs with concurrent nasal discharge and has demonstrated hyperemia and eosinophilic nasal cytology (Clercx et al. 2000). Intradermal skin testing has occasionally been employed in an attempt to identify a potential allergic stimulus for EBP but results have been equivocal.

Treatment

Dogs with EBP are often treated prophylactically for parasites or larval migration with fenbendazole (50 mg/kg/day for 14 days) while bacterial cultures are pending. Specific therapy for EBP requires the use of immunosuppressive doses of prednisone or prednisolone.

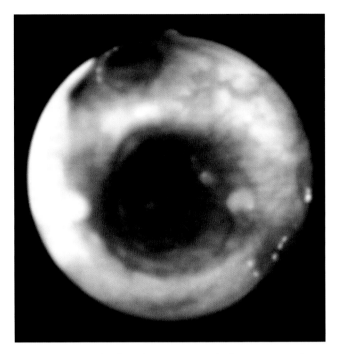

Figure 6.9.   Bronchoscopic image from the dog of Figure 6.8 reveals dramatic airway hyperemia and mild mucus accumulation.

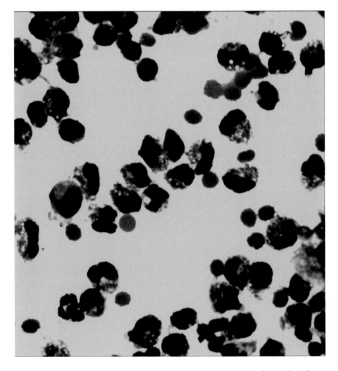

Figure 6.10.   Airway cytology from a dog with eosinophilic lung disease confirms the diagnosis.

If clinical signs diminish in the first 10–14 days, a gradual decrease in corticosteroid dose and lengthening of the dosing interval are recommended. Peripheral eosinophilia should resolve relatively quickly, and pulse oximetry or arterial blood gas analysis demonstrates improvements in oxygenation prior to resolution of radiographic infiltrates. If clinical signs do not respond to systemic steroids or side effects are dose limiting, use of inhaled steroids could be implemented (see Chapter 3).

Treatment with oral and/or inhaled corticosteroids generally requires 4–6 months of tapering therapy, and in rare instances, other immunosuppressive drugs such as cyclosporine may be required. Limiting exposure to irritants in the environment is wise. The utility of hyposensitization therapy in EBP has not been fully assessed.

Prognosis

Degranulation of eosinophils during bronchoscopy or tracheal wash can lead to bronchoconstriction or noncardiogenic pulmonary edema. This is manifest by decompensation and dramatic respiratory distress. Rapid confirmation of airway eosinophilia and administration of steroids can be life saving. Dogs with EBP generally respond to therapy; however, long-term treatment is often required to avoid relapses, and side effects of steroids can be significant.

Aspiration Pneumonia

Pathophysiology

Aspiration pneumonia is a serious and potentially life-threatening inflammatory and/or infectious lung process that occurs secondary to inhalation of gastric or oropharyngeal contents. Pulmonary injury results from chemical pneumonitis, inflammatory pulmonary responses, and development of bacterial pneumonia. Initially, aspiration of gastric acid alters surfactant function resulting in loss of surface tension and atelectasis. Injury to epithelial cells allows bacterial invasion and also exposes nerve endings between epithelial cells, resulting in bronchoconstriction. Resultant inflammation and infection increase mucus production causing airway obstruction and difficulty breathing. Ventilation/perfusion mismatching results in hypoxemia. Severe aspiration injury is associated with increased alveolocapillary permeability and development of acute respiratory distress syndrome due to noncardiogenic pulmonary edema (see Chapter 8).

Aspiration pneumonia is usually associated with a single underlying disease, but multiple predisposing factors may be found. Esophageal dysfunction, vomiting, neurologic disorders, laryngeal disease, and post anesthetic aspiration are identified most commonly (Kogan et al. 2008b).

History and signalment

Aspiration pneumonia appears to be much more common in dogs than in cats, and any age or breed may be affected because of the multitude of predisposing diseases that can result in aspiration pneumonia. Cough and increased respiratory effort are noted in more than half of cases. Generally the history will provide clues to the underlying disease process leading to aspiration, such as a recent anesthetic event, seizure, or vomiting episode; however, it is uncommon for the aspiration episode to be witnessed.

Physical examination

Abnormal lung sounds are found in over half of dogs with aspiration pneumonia, although half of these may have only harsh or loud lung sounds while the other half will have detectable crackles or wheezes. Normal lung sounds have been reported in 30% of dogs and approximately 10% had dampened lung sounds (Kogan et al. 2008a). Fever (temperature >39.2°C [>102.5°F]) or tachypnea (respiratory rate >30 breaths/minute) is relatively common but may be found in less than half of affected dogs.

The remainder of the physical examination is important for determining the underlying etiology of aspiration. Stridor over the larynx is suspicious for laryngeal disease, and some dogs may display reduced gag reflex associated with generalized neuromuscular disease. In such animals, complete neurologic assessment is warranted. Observing the animal eat is beneficial in detecting subtle abnormalities in pharyngeal or esophageal function, and thorough abdominal palpation can be helpful in determining the etiology of vomiting.

Diagnostic findings

Neutrophilia with a left shift is present in the majority of affected dogs, indicating a response to inflammation, and albumin is often mildly decreased, perhaps due to lung inflammation and vascular leakage. Pulse oximetry or arterial blood gas analysis should be performed when available to assess the degree of lung dysfunction because some dogs are markedly hypoxemic.

The classic radiographic description of aspiration pneumonia is an alveolar infiltrate in the cranioventral or middle lung lobe region; however, approximately 25% of dogs can have an interstitial infiltrate at the time of diagnosis. Aspiration into the right lung occurs in over 50% of cases while both sides of the lung are involved in 12% (Kogan et al. 2008a). The most commonly involved lung lobe is the right middle lobe (Figure 6.11), followed by the right cranial and the caudal segment of the left cranial lobe, and the cranial segment of the left cranial lung lobe, although any lung lobe can be involved, depending on the position of the animal at the time of aspiration.

Airway wash samples would be expected to reveal septic suppurative inflammation and various bacterial species, particularly enteric organisms and *Mycoplasma*, on culture; however, these samples are rarely obtained because of concerns about further aspiration following sedation for collection of airway fluid.

Treatment

Standard therapy for pneumonia is recommended. Although antibiotic administration is somewhat controversial because not all aspiration events are associated with infection, broad-spectrum agents are usually given for 3–4 weeks. Bronchodilators may be helpful in the acute stage of disease, particularly if expiratory effort or wheezing suggest bronchoconstriction. Maintenance of airway hydration with intravenous fluids is important. Although saline nebulization and coupage is usually recommended for patients with pneumonia, it is difficult to perform in recumbent patients and would not be recommended in those with vomiting disorders because of the potential to increase intra-abdominal pressure and augment vomiting. Corticosteroids are not routinely recommended despite the fact that an inflammatory response contributes to pulmonary injury.

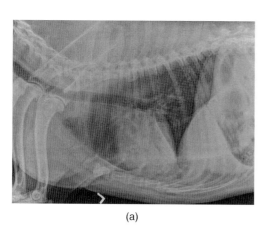
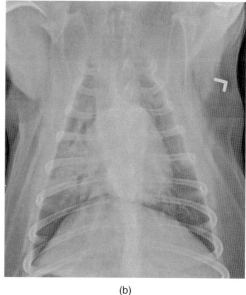

(a)   (b)

Figure 6.11. Right lateral (a) and dorsoventral (b) radiographs from a 12-year-old FS Labrador retriever with aspiration pneumonia, following unilateral arytenoid lateralization for treatment of laryngeal paralysis. Air bronchograms are visible in both views, primarily in the right middle lung lobe.

Animals that are not markedly hypoxemic or exhibiting dramatic respiratory effort can be maintained out of oxygen, because experimental evidence suggests that oxygen can enhance acid-induced injury. However, aspiration pneumonia can lead to acute respiratory distress syndrome (see Chapter 8), and in these patients, mechanical ventilation is often required.

Management of the primary disease responsible for aspiration is critical to avoid further aspiration and perpetuation of airway injury. Upright feeding and watering are important for animals with esophageal or laryngeal disease. Modification of the consistency of the diet should be instituted because some animals are better able to prehend and swallow kibble while others do well with meatball or slurry feeding.

Prognosis

In one study, over 75% of dogs with aspiration pneumonia survived, despite the presence of more than one predisposing disorder for aspiration (Kogan et al. 2008b). Interestingly, radiographic severity of disease and duration of hospitalization were not associated with overall survival rate.

Interstitial Lung Disease

Pathophysiology

Various pathologic forms of interstitial lung disease (ILD) have been described in dogs and cats, including idiopathic pulmonary fibrosis (defined histologically as usual interstitial pneumonia), cryptogenic fibrosing alveolitis, and bronchiolitis obliterans with organizing pneumonia. Some of these diseases are characterized by inflammation while in others, the interstitium is infiltrated by fibroblasts and there is collagen deposition, smooth muscle and alveolar epithelial metaplasia, and very little inflammation. The latter infiltrative form is termed idiopathic pulmonary fibrosis and has been described in the cat (Cohn et al. 2004). It is also the most common form of interstitial lung disease suspected in terrier-type dogs, although one histopathologic evaluation suggested that the syndrome is related to failure of collagenolysis (Norris et al. 2005).

In human medicine, interstitial lung disease has been reported secondary to infectious organisms (bacteria, viruses, or fungi), exposure to drugs (e.g., antibiotics or anti-arrhythmics agents) or inhaled toxins (e.g., paraquat), and in association with neoplasia. It is suspected that similar disorders can lead to ILD in dogs and cats because they are characterized by damage to the alveolar-capillary membrane. Epithelial cell activation and induction of inflammation followed by a dysregulated mesenchymal repair process lead to structural changes in the alveolar unit and dysfunctional gas exchange. Some dogs may be affected by concurrent bronchitis, which obscures the underlying lung disease. In the cat, coincident pulmonary neoplasia has been noted in 25% of cases (Cohn et al. 2004).

History and signalment

This disorder afflicts terriers (particularly West Highland white terriers) more commonly than other breeds and various types of cats. Animals are usually middle aged to older at the time of presentation, and generally, there is a chronic history of gradual deterioration in systemic health and exercise tolerance prior to the onset of tachypnea and eventual respiratory distress or failure. Occasionally, younger (2–5-year-old) large-breed dogs develop interstitial lung disease of unknown etiology, and severe signs are usually seen.

A dry, nonproductive cough may predominate in some animals, or owners may report loud respirations or rapid breathing. Systemic signs of lethargy, anorexia, and weight loss are relatively common, especially in cats. Severely affected animals may develop syncope due to hypoxemia or pulmonary hypertension.

Physical examination

Tachypnea can be dramatic in affected animals with respiratory rates of 100–150 breaths/minute in the absence of panting. The classic auscultatory finding is inspiratory crackles, which can be soft or loud, and are often present diffusely throughout all lung fields. Some animals may display only increased or loud bronchovesicular sounds, and expiratory wheezes may be apparent, either as part of the disease process or as a reflection of concurrent bronchitis. Animals with secondary pulmonary hypertension may develop a right-sided systolic murmur of tricuspid regurgitation or a split-second heart sound. The remainder of the physical examination is usually unremarkable.

Diagnostic findings

The minimum database is used to rule out concurrent systemic diseases. Laboratory findings of a neutrophilic leukocytosis and mild hyperproteinemia reflect chronic inflammation. Pulse oximetry (or arterial blood gas) is recommended to assess the degree of dysfunction because dramatic hypoxemia (P_aO_2 <50 mm Hg) can be seen in dogs.

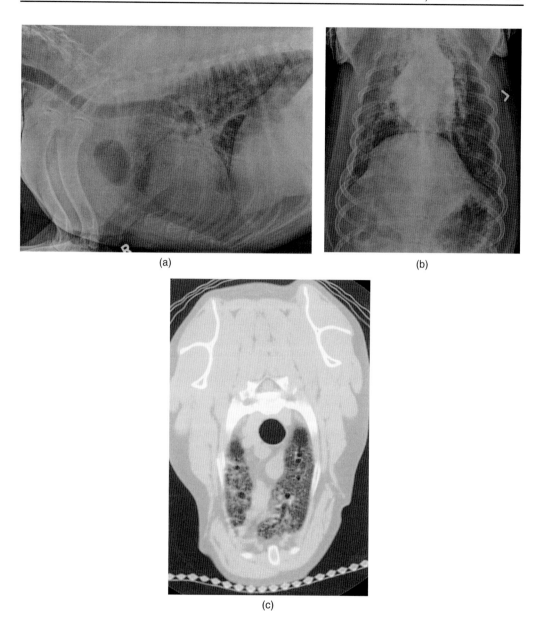

(a)   (b)

(c)

Figure 6.12.   Right lateral (a) and dorsoventral (b) radiographs of a 2-year-old MC Chesapeake Bay retriever reveal severe, diffuse miliary interstitial infiltrates throughout all lung lobes and mild perihilar lymphadenopathy. The right heart and pulmonary arteries are moderately enlarged. Computed tomography (c) demonstrates severe peribronchial and alveolar infiltrates throughout all lung lobes.

Thoracic radiographs in dogs typically show a generalized or diffuse mild, moderate, or severe, interstitial pattern that obscures visualization of the vasculature, and computed tomography can highlight the severity of the infiltrate (Figure 6.12). Moderate cardiomegaly is relatively common in dogs and is primarily right sided. Variable diffuse or patchy interstitial, bronchial and/or alveolar infiltrates are observed in cats, and radiographic changes are generally described as severe, with caudal lobes more prominently involved (Cohn et al.

2004). Additional findings include bronchiectasis or cavitated lesions (which could indicate concurrent neoplasia).

Airway sampling by tracheal wash or bronchoscopy can be performed as a less invasive alternative to lung biopsy, although a nonspecific increase in nondegenerate neutrophils and/or lymphocytes is typically seen. Epithelial dysplasia can be predominant finding. Definitive diagnosis of interstitial lung disease requires histopathologic evaluation of a lung sample obtained through thoracotomy, thoracoscopy, or key-hole lung biopsy. Preoperative computed tomography is recommended to identify the extent of parenchymal changes and to identify a site for lung biopsy or lobectomy because disease is often patchy in distribution. Histopathologic findings of alveolar septal fibrosis, type II pneumocyte hyperplasia, smooth muscle cell hyperplasia, and epithelial metaplasia can be locally extensive or diffuse.

Treatment

Unfortunately, treatment options are limited and fibrotic changes do not respond to anti-inflammatory therapy, although signs of concurrent bronchitis can be alleviated by oral or inhaled corticosteroids. Exposure to toxins and inhalation injury should be avoided, weight control is important, and a bronchodilator trial could be considered. In some animals, oxygen therapy at night can improve daytime activities (see Chapter 3). Alternate therapy remains under investigation pending further information regarding the etiology of disease.

Prognosis

Prognosis is guarded because no effective treatment has been recognized and because of the presence of concurrent pulmonary neoplasia in cats. Survival times vary from weeks to months. Some animals may develop pulmonary hypertension, which can be variably managed (see Chapter 8).

Neoplastic Lung Disease

Pathophysiology

The lung is a very common site for metastatic neoplasia from carcinomas or sarcomas and is also affected by primary neoplasia (adenocarcinoma, alveolar carcinoma, bronchoalveolar carcinoma, squamous cell carcinoma, and lymphosarcoma).

History and signalment

Primary and metastatic pulmonary neoplasia affects older animals most commonly. Clinical complaints may be indicative of respiratory disease and include cough, labored breathing, tachypnea, or hemoptysis, but in many cases (particularly in cats), nonrespiratory signs of anorexia and weight loss are reported. Cats may also be presented for lameness associated with digital metastasis from a primary pulmonary neoplasia (Gottfried et al. 2000).

Physical examination

Affected animals often display tachypnea associated with either neoplastic parenchymal infiltration or pleural effusion associated with neoplasia. Lung sounds can be harsh or

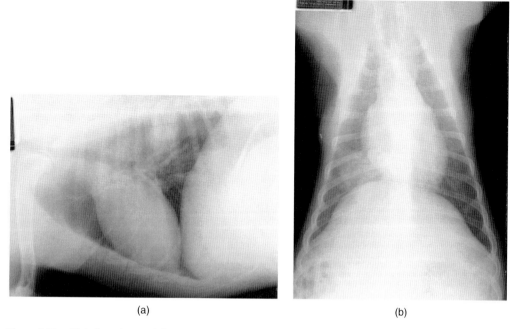

(a)   (b)

Figure 6.13.   Right lateral (a) and dorsoventral (b) radiographs from a 5-year-old MC Rhodesian Ridgeback with a primary lung tumor in the right caudal lung lobe. No obvious hilar lymphadenopathy or intrapulmonary metastases are visible on radiographs; however, a metastatic nodule was detected in the right middle lung lobe with computed tomography.

abnormal with parenchymal disease, or they may be muffled when lobar consolidation or pleural effusion is present. Some animals develop acute clinical signs if a neoplasm ruptures and results in pneumothorax. In those cases, lung sounds are absent dorsally and hyperresonanace might be detected.

Diagnostic findings

Primary pulmonary neoplasia is usually focal and appears as single- or multiple-mass lesions or as lobar consolidation (Figure 6.13). In the dog, the right caudal lung lobe is affected most commonly while the left caudal lobe is reportedly involved more often in cats. Bronchogenic carcinoma in the cat can have a cystic appearance on radiographs or computed tomography associated with tumor necrosis (Figure 6.14). A diffuse pulmonary infiltrative pattern can also be found, particularly when a primary lung tumor has undergone intrapulmonary metastasis.

Metastatic disease in the dog is often characterized radiographically by multiple, discrete, interstitial nodules of variable sizes (Figure 6.15), or a diffuse interstitial pattern can be seen (Figure 6.16). In the cat, ill-defined nodules or diffuse, patchy, mixed alveolar patterns are found most commonly (Forrest and Graybush 1998). In either species, pleural effusion may obscure visualization of a mass lesion.

Occasionally, intraluminal masses are visualized bronchoscopically (Figure 6.17) and a biopsy sample can be obtained to confirm the diagnosis by cytology or histopathology (Figure 6.18). A fine-needle aspirate of the lung can be obtained in the awake or sedated animal with or without ultrasound guidance (see Chapter 2).

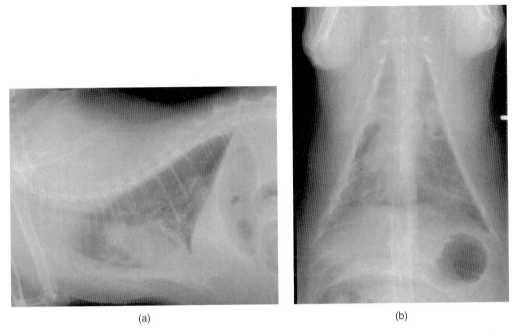

(a)   (b)

Figure 6.14. Right lateral (a) and dorsoventral (b) radiographs from a 12-year-old FS DLH with a primary lung in the caudal portion of the left cranial lung lobe and intrapulmonary metastases throughout the lung. Note the cavitated appearance of the primary lung mass and dilation of the bronchus.

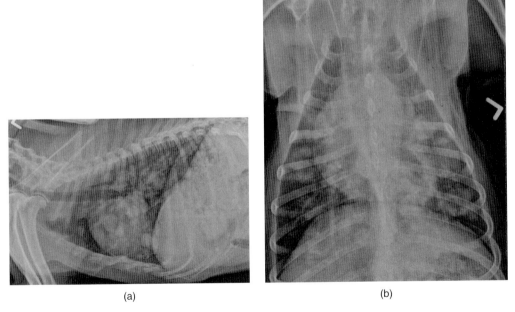

(a)   (b)

Figure 6.15. Pulmonary metastasis of a thyroid carcinoma in a 13-year-old FS English Shorthair Pointer. Variably sized nodules of soft tissue density are scattered throughout the lung parenchyma on the left lateral (a) and dorsoventral (b) views.

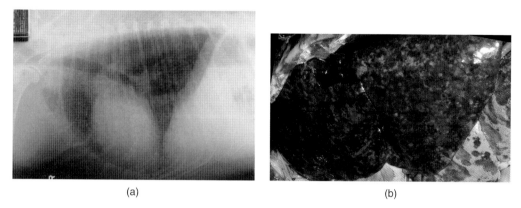

(a)   (b)

Figure 6.16. Right lateral radiograph (a) and gross necropsy findings (b) in a 10-year-old FS Standard Poodle with miliary pulmonary metastasis from a primary hemangiosarcoma.

Treatment

Surgical resection can be performed if primary or metastatic neoplasia affects a single lung lobe, or when multiple nodules are detected but less than three lung lobes are involved. No information is available on post operative chemotherapy for primary lung tumors in dogs or cats.

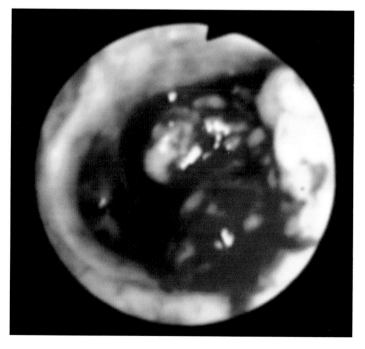

Figure 6.17. Bronchoscopic image from a 10-year-old MC DSH presented with a 2-month history of a dry cough and weight loss. A polypoid irregular bleeding mass can be seen partially obstructing a bronchus. Histopathology revealed a carcinoma combining properties of malignant epithelial and mesenchymal cells.

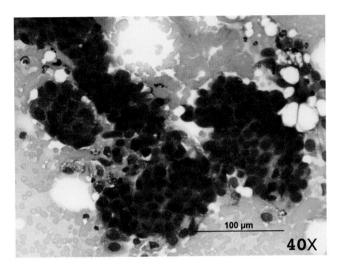

Figure 6.18. Cytology from a bronchoalveolar lavage sample in a 13-year-old MC Bassett Hound presented for chronic cough and hemoptysis. Characteristics of malignancy include a high nuclear/cytoplasmic ratio with some cells displaying marked anisocytosis and anisokaryosis with multiple large prominent nucleoli.

Prognosis

Prognosis depends on tumor histology as well as involvement of regional lymph nodes. In dogs treated with lobectomy for a solitary pulmonary mass, median survival for primary pulmonary neoplasia ranges from 8–20 months. In cats with histologically well-differentiated pulmonary tumors, median survival is 2 years while those with poorly differentiated neoplasms have <3 months, median survival (Hahn and McEntee 1998). Unfortunately, the majority of animals with primary pulmonary neoplasia have metastasis to bronchial lymph nodes, other lung lobes, pleura, skeletal muscle, skin, liver, spleen, or brain at the time of diagnosis.

References

Angus JC, Jang SS, Hirsh DC. Microbiologic study of transtracheal aspirates from dogs with suspected lower respiratory tract disease: 264 cases (1989–1995). J Am Vet Med Assoc. 1997; 210: 55–58.

Bart M, Guscetti F, Zurbriggen A, et al. Feline infectious pneumonia. A short literature review and a retrospective immunohistological study on the involvement of *Chlamydia* spp. and distemper virus. Vet J. 2000; 159: 220–230.

Clercx C, Peeters D, Snaps F, et al. Eosinophilic bronchopneumopathy in dogs. J Vet Int Med. 2000; 14: 282–291.

Clercx C, Peeters D, German AJ, et al. An immunologic investigation of canine eosinophilic bronchopneumopathy, J Vet Int Med. 2002: 16; 229–237.

Clercx C, Reichler I, Peeters D, et al. Rhinitis/bronchopneumonia syndrome in Irish wolfhounds. J Vet Int Med. 2003; 17: 843–849.

Cohn LA, Norris CR, Hawkins EC, et al. Identification and characterization of an idiopathic pulmonary fibrosis-like condition in cats. J Vet Int Med. 2004; 18: 632–641.

Forrest LJ, Graybush CA. Radiographic patterns of pulmonary metastasis in 25 cats. Vet Radiol Ultrasound. 1998; 39: 4–8.

Foster SF, Martin P, Allan GS, et al. Lower respiratory tract infections in cats: 21 cases (1995–2000). J Feline Med Surg. 2004; 6: 167–180.

Gottfried SD, Popovitch CA, Goldschmidt MH, Schelling C. Bronchogenic carcinoma and metastasis to the digits in cats. J Am Anim Hosp Assoc. 2000; 36: 501–509.

Greene RT, Troy GC. Coccidioidomycosis in 48 cats: A retrospective study. J Vet Int Med. 1995; 9: 86–91.

Hahn KA, McEntee MF. Prognosis factors for survival in cats after removal of a primary lung tumor: 21 cases (1979–1994). Vet Surg. 1998; 27: 307–311.

Kogan DA, Johnson LR, Jandrey KE, Pollard RE. Clinicopathologic and radiographic findings in dogs with aspiration pneumonia: 88 cases (2004–2006). J Am Vet Med Assoc. 2008a; 233: 1642–1747.

Kogan DA, Johnson LR, Sturges BK, et al. Etiology and clinical outcome in dogs with aspiration pneumonia: 88 cases (2004–2006). J Am Vet Med Assoc. 2008b; 233: 1748–1755.

Legendre AM, Rohrbach BW, Toal RL, et al. Treatment of blastomycosis with itraconazole in 112 dogs. J Vet Int Med. 1996; 10: 365–371.

Lobetti R. Common variable immunodeficiency in miniature dachshunds affected with *Pneumonocystis carinii* pneumonia. J Vet Diag Invest. 2000; 12: 39–45.

Murphy ST, Ellison GW, McKiernan BC, et al. Pulmonary lobectomy in the management of pneumonia in dogs: 59 cases (1972–1994). J Am Vet Med Assoc. 1997; 210: 235–239.

Neath PJ, Brockman DJ, King LG. Lung lobe torsion in dogs: 22 cases (1981–1999). J Am Vet Med Assoc. 2000; 217: 1041–1044.

Norris AJ, Naydan DK, Wilson DW. Interstitial lung disease in West Highland White Terriers. Vet Pathol. 2005; 42: 35–41.

Peeters D, Peters IR, Clercx C, Day MJ. Real-time RT-PCR quantification of mRNA encoding cytokines, CC chemokines and CCR3 in bronchial biopsies from dogs with eosinophilic bronchopneumopathy. Vet Immunol Immunopathol. 2006; 110: 65–77.

Radhakrishnan A, Drobatz KJ, Culp WT, et al. Community-acquired infectious pneumonia in puppies: 65 cases (1993–2002). J Am Vet Med Assoc. 2007; 230: 1493–1497.

Shubitz LE, Butkiewicz CD, Dial SM, Lindan CP. Incidence of *Coccidioides* infection among dogs residing in a region in which the organism is endemic. J Am Vet Med Assoc. 2005; 226: 1846–1850.

Simons FA, Vennema H, Rofina JE, et al. A mRNA PCR for the diagnosis of feline infectious peritonitis. J Virol Methods. 2005; 124: 111–116.

Spector D, Legendre AM, Wheat J, et al. Antigen and antibody testing for the diagnosis of blastomycosis in dogs. J Vet Int Med. 2008; 22: 839–843.

Watson PJ, Wotton P, Eastwood J, et al. Immunoglobulin deficiency in Cavalier King Charles Spaniels with *Pneumocystis* pneumonia. J Vet Int Med. 2006; 20: 523–527.

Pleural and Mediastinal Disease

7

Structural Disorders

Pneumothorax

Pathophysiology

Entrance of air into the pleural cavity results in positive intrapleural pressure that causes collapse of the lungs with a subsequent drop in venous return and cardiac output. The most common cause of pneumothorax is blunt or penetrating chest trauma. Esophageal perforation or foreign body migration can also lead to pneumothorax. Spontaneous pneumothorax results from rupture of an emphysematous bulla, pleural bleb, neoplasm, *Paragonimus kellicotti* cyst, or of a necrotic or abscessed lung lobe. Multiple lung lobes can be involved depending on the disease process, and cranial lobes are affected most commonly in spontaneous pneumothorax.

A specific form of pneumothorax is a tension pneumothorax, where a piece of pulmonary tissue or pleura acts as a ball-valve, allowing passage of air into the pleural space during inspiration with inhibition of escape of air via the same pathway. In this situation, air continues to accumulate in the pleural space, leading to a continual rise in intrapleural pressure and circulatory collapse.

History and signalment

Any age or breed of dog or cat can be affected. Spontaneous pneumothorax associated with underlying lung disease appears to be more common in middle-aged large-breed dogs, and in one study, Siberian Huskies were overrepresented (Puerto et al. 2002). It is less common in cats but can occur secondary to chronic bronchial disease. The most common cause of pneumothorax in dogs and cats is trauma, from a car collision, falling from a height, or a thoracic bite wound. In suburban and rural areas, migrating grass awns are also implicated as a cause for pneumothorax. Iatrogenic pneumothorax occurs secondary to barotrauma during anesthesia, endotracheal tube injury, fine-needle lung aspiration, or bronchoscopy.

The primary clinical complaints associated with pneumothorax are difficulty breathing or tachypnea, and these are usually seen immediately after the injury or rupture of a pulmonary lesion. Some cases with spontaneous pneumothorax may lack a history of signs referable to the respiratory tract, and will display chronic, nonspecific signs of lethargy and anorexia prior to development of worsening respiratory difficulty.

Physical examination

Accumulation of air in the pleural space leads to rapid and shallow breathing, and lung sounds are usually difficult to discern. Air in the pleural space will rise, leading to an absence of breath sounds dorsally and hyperresonance on percussion. Animals involved in traumatic episodes should be closely evaluated for additional injuries including broken ribs, diaphragmatic hernia, and pulmonary contusions.

Diagnostic findings

Pneumothorax is usually bilateral and is recognized by an absence of lung parenchyma and pulmonary vasculature in the periphery of the lung on thoracic radiographs. The heart is usually lifted off the sternum on the lateral view (Figure 7.1). While pneumothorax is

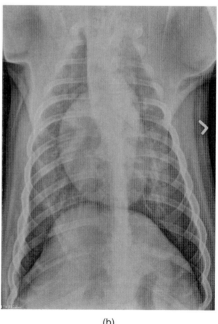
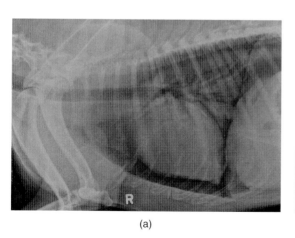

(a) (b)

Figure 7.1. Right lateral (a) and dorsoventral (b) radiographs from a 6-year-old MI Labrador Retriever with spontaneous pneumothorax.

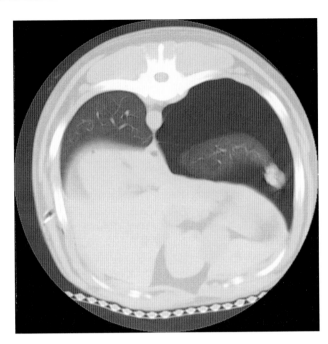

Figure 7.2. Computed tomographic slice through the caudal thorax in the dog from Figure 7.1 illustrates a soft tissue structure in the distal portion of the right caudal lung lobe. Histopathology revealed a pulmonary adenocarcinoma.

readily apparent on chest radiographs, the underlying lesion is often not visible, particularly when bullous lung disease or pleural blebs are the cause of pneumothorax. Cross-sectional imaging with computed tomography (CT) improves definition of lung regions (Figure 7.2), and when sufficient lung expansion can be obtained to alleviate atelectasis, it can be helpful in identifying diseased regions (Au et al. 2006).

For animals from the Midwest or Gulf States or those that may have been exposed to *Paragonimus*, a trematode that employs snails and crustaceans as intermediate hosts, a fecal sedimentation or zinc sulfate centrifugation–flotation should be performed. In dogs, thoracic radiographs may show multiple thin-walled cavitated cysts, while in the cat, thick-walled granulomatous lesions and pleural involvement are more typical.

Treatment

Thoracocentesis should be performed when pneumothorax is suspected and may be required as a life-saving procedure prior to radiographic confirmation of pneumothorax in order to resolve respiratory distress. With traumatic pneumothorax, a single chest tap and alleviation of respiratory distress through sedation and administration of oxygen will often restore pleural integrity and result in cure. If *Paragonimus* is diagnosed, praziquantel (25 mg/kg PO TID for 3 days) or fenbendazole (50 mg/kg/day for 2 weeks) have been recommended as effective (Bowman et al. 1991), although surgical resection of the diseased lung region is also required.

If air continues to accumulate within the pleural space after several chest taps, placement of a chest tube is required (see Chapter 3). Generally, spontaneous pneumothorax and tension pneumothorax will require placement of a chest tube and constant thoracic drainage to resolve air leakage. Because underlying lung disease is often present with spontaneous pneumothorax, surgical intervention is usually required to avoid recurrence. When pneumothorax does not resolve within 3–5 days or if parenchymal lesions causing pneumothorax are visualized on radiographs, an exploratory thoracotomy should be performed. Median sternotomy is usually preferred to allow full exploration of the lungs.

Prognosis

Traumatic pneumothorax generally has a good prognosis if traumatic myocarditis and pulmonary contusions do not complicate the presentation. The prognosis for spontaneous pneumothorax depends on the underlying disease responsible for air leakage. Surgical resection of the affected area is associated with an excellent outcome in most dogs with emphysematous lung disease, foreign body pleuropneumonia, or *Paragonimus* infection.

Pneumomediastinum

Pathophysiology

Pneumomediastinum is an accumulation of air around the structures in the cranial mediastinum (carotid arteries, vagosympathetic trunk, trachea, esophagus, and cranial vena cava). It occurs most commonly from endotracheal tube injury or overinflation of the cuff, traumatic jugular venipuncture, or a transtracheal wash. It is also associated with trauma from a dog fight or from overventilation during anesthesia. It can occur with bronchial, tracheal, or alveolar rupture when air tracks along fascial planes to reach the mediastinum.

History and signalment

Any age dog or cat can be affected. Usually a history of trauma or iatrogenic injury is present immediately prior to the onset of signs or within a week of presentation. In cats, a recent dental procedure is often found in the history. Often no clinical signs are noted, and pneumomediastinum is an incidental finding on radiographs, following traumatic venipuncture or tracheal wash. In more severely affected animals, tachypnea, respiratory distress, or collapse associated with pneumothorax may result. Owners may detect subcutaneous emphysema concentrated over the neck, thorax, and head.

Physical examination

Mild, moderate, or severe subcutaneous emphysema may be detected. When pneumothorax is present, tachypnea is often evident, and lung sounds are absent dorsally.

Diagnostic testing

Diagnosis is based on radiography. Pneumomediastinum is evident when outer borders of the trachea, esophagus, carotid arteries, aorta, and azygous veins are visible because of contrast with mediastinal air. Subcutaneous emphysema may be detected over the trunk (Figure 7.3). If tracheal rupture is suspected, tracheoscopy can occasionally be helpful in locating the lesion; however, surgical exploration is usually required.

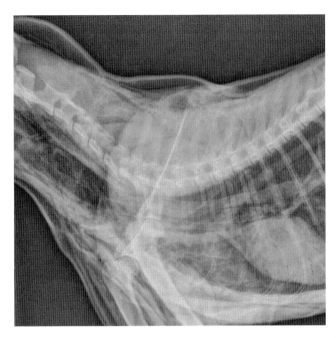

Figure 7.3.   Right lateral radiograph from an 18-month-old FS DSH that had been anesthetized 2 weeks previously and developed subcutaneous emphysema and pneumomediastinum.

Treatment

Generally no specific treatment is required and air will resorb within 10–20 days. Concurrent pneumothorax requires thoracocentesis. If respiratory distress is present, oxygen therapy is helpful for reducing the work of breathing, and judicious use of sedatives to reduce stress is important. If tachypnea or respiratory effort increases, surgical repair of the lesion is necessary.

Prognosis

Prognosis is usually excellent for resolution of disease. When pneumomediastinum is detected, restraint methods and diagnostic techniques should be reviewed for predisposing features that might have led to airway injury. In cats, <3 mL of air is generally required to inflate the cuff of an endotracheal tube sufficiently.

Diaphragmatic Hernia

Pathophysiology

Blunt trauma to the abdomen increases intracavitary pressure leading to rupture of the muscular portion of the diaphragm and herniation of abdominal organs into the thoracic cavity. The liver is involved most frequently, followed by the small intestine and stomach. The lungs collapse because of loss of contact between visceral and parietal pleura and from compression by abdominal organs. Fluid accumulation in the thorax due to hemorrhage or transudation from the organ surface further restricts lung expansion and worsens oxygenation and ventilation. Animals with herniation of the stomach into the chest cavity can suffer rapid decompensation if aerophagia results in continual expansion of the stomach. The space occupying effect of gastric dilation augments lung compression, with a decrease in venous return and subsequently cardiac output.

History and signalment

Affected animals may have a history of recent trauma within the past several hours or may have experienced injury years in the past. Most dogs and cats are young (3–4 years) in age. Clinical signs are usually respiratory in origin and include tachypnea and difficulty breathing, but some animals are presented for acute or chronic vomiting or regurgitation associated with gastrointestinal obstruction or strangulation. Still others may develop progressive exercise intolerance or respiratory difficulty associated with gradual accumulation of pleural fluid.

Physical examination

Animals with organ herniation or pleural effusion often have muffling of heart and lung sounds ventrally or on one side of the chest. When herniation has been present for >24–48 hours, intestinal borborygmi may be auscultated over the thorax (Figure 7.4). Occasionally,

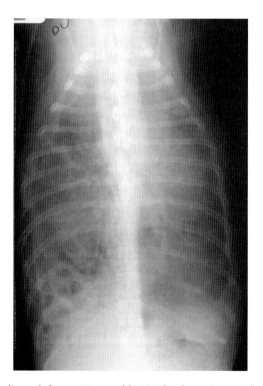

Figure 7.4. Dorsoventral radiograph from a 12-year-old MC Labrador retriever with exercise intolerance reveals gastrointestinal loops in the right hemithorax. Physical examination findings included absent lung sounds in the right hemithorax and the presence of gastrointestinal sounds.

abdominal palpation may reveal an absence of contents. Traumatic injury to other structures in the thorax, abdomen, or skeleton can be found in 25–40% of cases, and a complete physical examination should be performed to detect findings consistent with traumatic myocarditis, urinary system rupture, rib fractures, or orthopedic injuries (Gibson et al. 2005).

Diagnostic findings

Thoracic and abdominal radiographs can usually confirm the diagnosis of a diaphragmatic hernia; however, if pleural effusion is present, thoracocentesis and repeat radiographs may be required to allow definition of the diaphragmatic silhouette and thoracic structures. Chronic cases are often more difficult to diagnose radiographically. A barium series can confirm the presence of intestines in the thoracic cavity or provide better definition of the position of the liver or small intestines, and ultrasound can occasionally be helpful. CT and/or exploratory surgery may be required for confirmation of the diagnosis.

Treatment

Surgical repair of the diaphragm is indicated, and artificial ventilation must be provided once the abdominal cavity has been opened. Cases with stomach herniation generally represent a surgical emergency because respiratory difficulty causes aerophagia, progressive stomach distention, and further respiratory compromise. Standard stabilization methods with intravenous fluid support and withdrawal of pleural fluid prior to anesthesia are important. Oxygenation, ventilation, and cardiac rhythm must be monitored carefully throughout the procedure.

Prognosis

Improvements in anesthetic drugs, monitoring, and assisted ventilation have vastly improved response to surgery. Diaphragmatic hernia repair is associated with an 80–90% survival rate (Gibson et al. 2005), regardless of whether the hernia is acute or chronic in nature and regardless of the time between admission and surgery. Owners should be aware that additional surgery might be required to repair soft tissue or orthopedic injuries that are not as life-threatening as the diaphragmatic hernia.

Infectious Disorders

Pyothorax

Pathophysiology

The etiology of pyothorax is often not determined. Bacteria can gain entry into the pleural space through a bite wound, penetrating injury, foreign body inhalation, direct puncture of the chest wall, or via esophageal rupture. Less commonly, bacteria can spread to the pleura from a pulmonary infection or hematogenously. Iatrogenic pyothorax results when aseptic technique is breached during thoracocentesis. The anaerobic environment within the pleural space promotes growth of various types of bacteria.

History and signalment

Pyothorax most commonly occurs in young, outdoor animals. Large-breed or hunting dogs and cats from multicat households are affected more commonly. Owners may seek veterinary attention primarily for respiratory signs but many affected animals have more prominent systemic signs of weight loss, anorexia, inactivity, and exercise intolerance. Clinical signs may be present for days to months before presentation.

Physical examination

Pyothorax is anticipated to result in a rapid shallow breathing pattern; however, both the rate and amount of fluid accumulation influence the severity of respiratory difficulty, and respiratory rate can be only mildly elevated in some cases. Fever may or may not be present at the time of presentation. Muffled heart and lung sounds are expected ventrally, although pyothorax can affect a single side of the thorax when the proteinaceous fluid occludes fenestrae in the mediastinum to create noncommunicating halves to the thorax. This could result in unilateral absence of lung sounds. Careful physical inspection of the thoracic wall may reveal recent or healed bite wounds.

Diagnostic findings

Hematology usually shows mild anemia and leukocytosis characterized by neutrophilia and monocytosis. Increased serum globulin is a nonspecific indicator of chronicity. Thoracic radiographs reveal unilateral or bilateral pleural effusion with obscuring of the cardiac silhouette and diaphragm, scalloping of ventral lung margins, and blunting of costophrenic angles (Figure 7.5). Evidence of a foreign body or a consolidated lung lobe is occasionally present. Thoracic ultrasound can be helpful in revealing flocculent or viscous pleural fluid and can sometimes detect lobar consolidation or a foreign body.

The initial step in confirming a diagnosis of pyothorax is to perform a chest tap (see Chapter 2). Cytologic analysis reveals an exudative fluid (high protein and high cell count) comprised primarily of degenerate neutrophils. Intracellular bacteria can be observed in up to 91% of cats and 68% of dogs (Walker et al. 2000) (Figure 7.6). A Gram stain can provide information on the type of bacteria present and improves choice of antibiotics while cultures are pending. Both aerobic and anaerobic cultures should be requested on a pleural exudate because mixed bacteria are usually found (Table 7.1). Note that a special transport medium may be required to obtain an accurate result for anaerobic bacteria.

Treatment

Successful treatment usually requires placement of uni- or bilateral chest tubes (see Chapter 3) and thoracic lavage with warm saline (10–20 mL/kg BID–QID). Addition of heparin to the lavage fluid (1500 units/100 mL) can reduce adhesions and promote drainage. The fluid is left in the chest cavity for 1 hour and then aspirated. The patient resorbs 10–25% of the fluid. Broad-spectrum antibiotics that are active against both aerobes and anaerobes

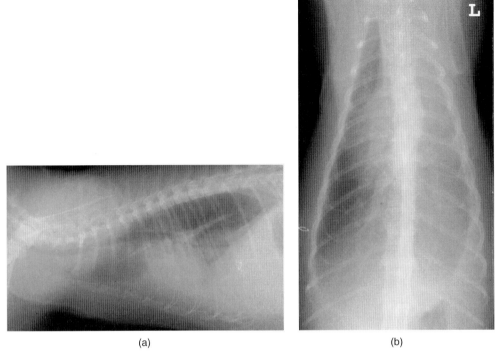

(a)   (b)

Figure 7.5. Right lateral (a) and dorsoventral (b) radiographs from a 10-year-old MC DMH presented for anorexia and weight loss. Physical examination revealed dampened heart and lung sounds ventrally, and radiographs confirmed the presence of pleural fluid.

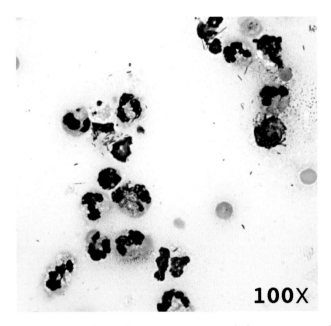

Figure 7.6. Pleural fluid cytology from the cat shown in Figure 7.5 reveals degenerate neutrophils and intracellular bacteria consistent with pyothorax.

Table 7.1. Organisms commonly identified in animals with pyothorax (Walker et al. 2000)

	Dog	Cat
Aerobes		
Enteric organisms—*Escherichia coli, Klebsiella, Enterobacter*	6/47: 22%	1/45: 4%
Nonenteric organisms—*Pasteurella, Acinetobacter, Pseudomonas*	10/47: 37%	19/45: 70%
Actinomyces	5/47: 19%	4/45: 15%
Anaerobes		
Peptostreptococcus	18/47: 27%	17/45: 20%
Bacteroides	17/47: 25%	20/45: 24%
Fusobacterium	14/47: 21%	14/45: 17%
Porphyromonas	6/47: 9%	10/45: 12%

are administered systemically. Anaerobic coverage should be provided even if cultures are negative. Penicillins and cephalosporins are commonly used alone or in combination with a fluoroquinolone. Trimethoprim sulfonamide is often employed if infection with *Nocardia* spp. is suspected. There is no advantage to adding antibiotics to the lavage fluid because the primary route of exposure of the pleura to antibiotics is through the systemic circulation.

Each day before instituting thoracic lavage, fluid is extracted from the thorax to evaluate the number and type of cells present and to check for the presence or absence of bacteria. Successful therapy is indicated by a reduction in cell numbers and decline in intracellular bacteria over several days of treatment. Medical therapy can take 3–7 days to be effective. Chest radiographs or ultrasound reevaluated as indicated to detect a mass lesion or foreign body. Prior to removal of the chest tube, a fluid sample should be submitted for aerobic and anaerobic culture to ensure successful resolution of infection.

Thoracotomy is required to remove a foreign body or to debride necrotic tissue. Surgical exploration is indicated when new radiographic findings are detected or if cell numbers or bacteria rise despite lavage and drainage therapy. Preoperative CT can help localize disease.

For owners lacking sufficient funds for hospitalization and treatment, consideration can be given to conservative medical management. One study reported successful management of 15 dogs with pyothorax by use of a single chest drainage and antibiotics (ampicillin TID with metronidazole BID most commonly) for >6 weeks (Johnson and Martin 2007). The risk of persistent infection must be communicated to the client if this mode of therapy is chosen.

Prognosis

The debate regarding medical versus surgical treatment of pyothorax is difficult to resolve since surgery is often delayed until medical therapy has failed or is undertaken because an obvious need for surgical intervention is noted, such as a foreign body. Success of therapy varies; however, when aggressive medical or surgical treatment is pursued, resolution is reported in 60–100% of cases. Early discontinuation of antibiotics can result in recurrent infection, and chronic pyothorax can be associated with constrictive pleuritis.

Mediastinitis

Pathophysiology

Mediastinitis can result from involvement of the mediastinum by infection with any fungal organism (see Chapter 6), by bacteria directly inoculated through the thorax or entering via esophageal or tracheal injury, or from spirocercosis, a worm that lives in the esophagus or stomach of the dog and causes neoplastic transformation of the tissue. *Spirocerca* has a worldwide distribution but is found more often in warm climates, and disease appears to occur most commonly in Israel. A dog becomes infected with *Spirocerca lupi* by eating a coprophagous beetle intermediate host or an animal that has eaten the beetle. The larvae gain access to the circulation and travel to the aorta where they enter the esophagus. Adult worms (5–7 cm in length) live inside nodules in the esophagus. Rupture of the nodule can result in mediastinitis, although usually infection either is subclinical or results in neoplastic transformation of tissue.

History and signalment

Outdoor dogs and dogs that hunt are more likely to be exposed to injury and also to carriers of *Spirocerca*. Young, outdoor dogs are also those more likely to develop fungal infection. Esophageal disease related to injury or spirocercosis generally results in signs of difficulty swallowing or regurgitation. Esophageal rupture is associated with acute onset of pain, labored respirations, and tachypnea.

Physical examination

Fever is expected with systemic fungal infections and with bacterial infection. The respiratory pattern is altered depending on the type and location of infection. Large mass lesions can compress the trachea and result in inspiratory obstruction. If pleural effusion develops secondary to a mass effect in the thorax, tachypnea would be expected. Depending on the level of lung or pleural involvement, abnormal lung sounds may be auscultated. In cats and small dogs, it may be more difficult to compress the cranial thorax due to the presence of a mass lesion. When a mass lesion puts pressure on the large vessels in the cranial mediastinum, subcutaneous edema may develop in the head and front legs (cranial vena cava syndrome).

Diagnostic testing

Radiographs reveal a mass effect within the cranial or caudal mediastinum. Spirocercosis most typically results in a caudal mediastinal mass; aortic mineralization or spondylitis in the caudal thorax may also be detected (Dvir et al. 2001). Diagnosis is confirmed by finding small, elongated nematode eggs in a fecal flotation or by documenting nodular lesions within the esophagus using radiography or endoscopy.

Ultrasound of cranial mediastinal masses is recommended to determine whether the mass lesion is cystic or solid, and to determine vascularity. Cytology of an aspirate can confirm neoplasia, and fungal or bacterial infection. Aerobic and anaerobic culture of aspirated material is recommended when bacterial infection is suspected because *Bacteroides* spp. are often involved in infection.

Treatment

Bacterial mediastinitis represents an encapsulated abscess. Surgical drainage and use of antibiotics with good spectrum against oral and gastrointestinal flora is indicated.

Spirocerca can be eliminated with various antihelminthics including fenbendazole and albendazole although long-term therapy with ivermectin or milbemycin oxime may be needed. Ivermectin should not be used in collie-type dogs.

Prognosis

If surgery is required to repair the esophagus or to remove a large helminth granuloma, prognosis is guarded for recovery. Development of neoplasia secondary to spirocercosis is a recognized complication that can result in death due to primary or metastatic disease.

Neoplastic Disorders

Pathophysiology

The most common tumor to affect the pleural surface primarily and cause pleural effusion is mesothelioma, and this is relatively rare in veterinary patients. Thoracic effusion due to neoplasia is more commonly associated with tumors that metastasize to the lungs and cause pleural effusion through lymphatic obstruction or altered vascular permeability. Mediastinal masses can be associated with effusion through vascular obstruction or fluid exudation from the tumor. Thymoma or lymphosarcoma are encountered in the cranioventral region, heart base tumor (chemodectoma), ectopic thyroid neoplasia, or lymphadenopathy can be found craniodorsally, and in the perihilar region, lymphadenopathy or heart base tumors can be identified. Neoplastic mass lesions must be distinguished from a granuloma or an abscess.

History and signalment

Neoplastic processes, both primary and metastatic, usually affect middle-aged to older animals. The exception is mediastinal lymphoma in the cat, which appears to have a predilection for young (<2 years of age) Siamese cats that are FeLV negative (Louwerens et al. 2005). Clinical complaints associated with malignant pleural effusion are usually respiratory difficulty while those associated with mediastinal masses are often related to compression of adjacent structures by a mass lesion. Impingement on the trachea leads to labored respiration (on inspiration and/or expiration) while compression of the esophagus results in dysphagia. Historical features in animals with thymoma might include signs associated with the paraneoplastic syndrome of myasthenia gravis such as muscle weakness, esophageal dysfunction, or collapse.

Physical examination

Pleural effusion leads to a restrictive pattern of respiration with increased respiratory rate. Alternately, a compressive mediastinal mass can result in obstructed breathing with prolonged inspiration and increased effort. Pleural effusion or a cranial mediastinal mass can lead to decreased thoracic compressibility. Obstruction of venous return by a mediastinal

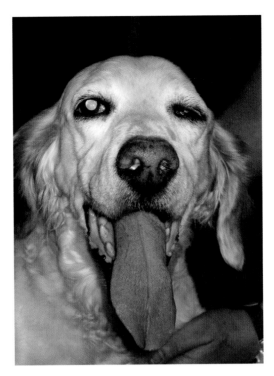

Figure 7.7. This 13-year-old FS English Setter demonstrates ptosis, enophthalmos, protrusion of third eyelid, and miosis OS consistent with Horner's syndrome on the left.

mass can lead to cranial vena cava syndrome with edema of the head, neck, and front limbs. Horner's syndrome (miosis, enophthalmos, and ptosis) (Figure 7.7) or stridor associated with laryngeal paralysis can occur when nerve transmission is interrupted by a mediastinal mass.

Diagnostic findings

Mesothelioma is anticipated to result in pleural effusion and mass lesions are generally not visible on radiographs. Pleural effusion cytology is often difficult to interpret in such cases because reactive mesothelial cells are encountered with a number of pleural disease processes. CT can sometimes identify lesions and will help direct surgical biopsies.

Animals with metastatic neoplasia may show evidence of nodular infiltrates or lymphadenopathy on radiographs after an effusion has been removed or on ultrasound.

Thoracic radiographic features of a mediastinal mass include dorsal deviation of the trachea and widening of the mediastinum (Figure 7.8). Pleural effusion may or may not be present. Thoracic ultrasound is useful for identifying characteristics of mediastinal mass lesions and can guide aspiration for cytology. Pleural fluid cytology is often diagnostic for neoplasia, and flow cytometry and polymerase chain reaction for antigen receptor rearrangement can be helpful in distinguishing thymoma from lymphoma (Lana et al. 2006).

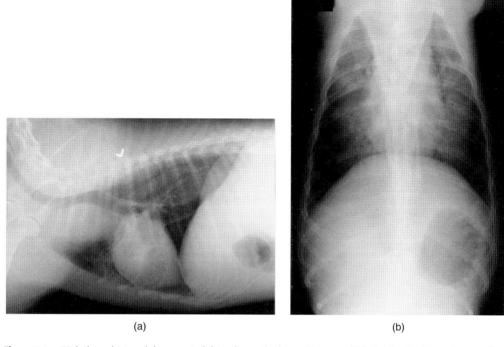

(a)   (b)

Figure 7.8. Right lateral (a) and dorsoventral (b) radiographs from a 3-year-old FS Golden Retriever. A mass effect in the mediastinum results in elevation of the trachea on the lateral view and widening of the mediastinum on the dorsoventral view.

Treatment

Protocols using various combinations of drugs including cyclophosphamide, vincristine, cytosine arabinoside, L-asparaginase, mitoxantrone, and prednisolone are recommended rather than single agent therapy for treating mediastinal lymphoma. Surgical resection is required for thymoma. No specific treatment is available for mesothelioma, although intracavitary cisplatin could be considered.

Prognosis

One study of lymphoma in the cat reported a median survival time of 9 months with 49% survival rate at 1 year with cyclophosphamide, vincristine, and prednisolone (Teske et al. 2002). Pleural effusion associated with primary pulmonary neoplasia, mesothelioma, or metastatic neoplasia carries a grave prognosis.

Miscellaneous Disorders

Pleural effusive diseases are categorized by the amount of protein in the fluid and cell count (see Chapter 2). After this initial staging, specific diagnostic tests are indicated to determine the most likely etiology of the effusion.

Hydrothorax

Pathophysiology

Hydrothorax refers to a low-protein fluid with low cellularity that accumulates within the thorax due to disturbance in Starling forces, the hydrostatic and oncotic pressures of the interstitial and vascular spaces (see the Starling equation—Equation 7.1). Hydrostatic pressure elevation associated with right-sided heart failure generally results in production of a modified transudate. Conditions that lead to loss of plasma oncotic pressure from low albumin result in transudative hydrothorax. This most commonly results from gastrointestinal loss of albumin due to lymphangiectasia, inflammatory bowel disease, or intestinal lymphoma, from protein losing nephropathy due to amyloidosis or glomerulonephritis, or from hypoalbuminemia associated with liver failure.

$$J_v = K_f[(P_c - P_i) - \sigma (\pi_c - \pi_i)] \tag{7.1}$$

where J_v is the net fluid movement, K_f is the filtration coefficient, P_c is the hydrostatic pressure in the capillary, P_i is the hydrostatic pressure in the interstitium, π_c is the oncotic pressure in the capillary, π_i is the oncotic pressure in the interstitium, and σ is the reflection coefficient.

History and signalment

The primary clinical complaints associated with hydrothorax are related to restriction of lung expansion due to fluid accumulation between the lung and chest wall. Clinical signs associated with the primary disease process responsible for hypoalbuminemia may predominate over those associated with fluid accumulation. Gastrointestinal disease may cause obvious signs of vomiting and diarrhea or may be associated with weight loss alone. Liver failure can also result in these signs and may be accompanied by neurologic signs associated with hepatic encephalopathy or bleeding due to loss of clotting factors. Glomerulonephritis is often clinically silent until renal insufficiency develops.

Physical examination

Animals with hydrothorax usually display a rapid, shallow breathing pattern, and pleural effusion should result in dampening of lung and heart sounds ventrally. Concurrent ascites is found in some patients; however, accumulation of fluid in the subcutaneous space is rare. Careful attention to the remainder of the physical examination is indicated to determine the underlying cause of hydrothorax. Infiltrative gastrointestinal disease should be suspected if diffusely thickened bowel loops are palpated; however, lymphangiectasia does not often result in palpable abnormalities. A palpably small liver may suggest liver failure; however, this is a very subjective finding.

Diagnostic testing

When hydrothorax is discovered, a systematic work-up is required to determine the underlying cause. A complete blood count may show lymphopenia suggestive of lymphangiectasia. When hypoalbuminemia is noted on the chemistry panel, and hypoglobulinemia is also found, abdominal ultrasound should be performed and gastrointestinal biopsies should be considered. If only low albumin is noted, a urinalysis should be evaluated for proteinuria. If a urine protein–creatinine ratio greater than 1 is detected in an animal with a negative urine culture, primary renal disease should be investigated in the presence or absence of azotemia. A tick panel, heartworm test, abdominal ultrasound, and possible kidney biopsy may be required to make the diagnosis. If low albumin is noted in conjunction with low blood urea nitrogen, low cholesterol, and low glucose, primary liver disease should be considered. Bile acids and abdominal ultrasound should then be pursued to rule out a portosystemic shunt.

A colloid osmotic/oncotic pressure (COP) can be measured to assess the magnitude of disruption in Starling forces. Normal values are 21–25 mm Hg in the dog and 23–25 mm Hg in the cat.

Treatment

Animals in respiratory distress due to accumulation of fluid should have sufficient pleural fluid removed to improve respirations; however, excessively rapid removal of fluid can theoretically lead to reexpansion pulmonary edema. Treatment of the underlying disease and elevation of albumin should result in a rise in COP and resolution of fluid accumulation. In some cases, administration of plasma (6–10 mL/kg), hetastarch (1–2 mL/kg/hour of 6 g/100 mL solution), or potentially concentrated human albumin can raise oncotic pressure sufficiently to alleviate fluid accumulation temporarily. Side effects include fever, fluid overload, or hypersensitivity reaction with plasma, coagulopathy with dextrans, and coagulopathy, hypersensitivity, or anaphylactic-like reactions with human albumin. In addition, delayed immune-type reactions to human albumin are suspected.

Prognosis

Prognosis depends on the underlying cause of disease. Unfortunately, the primary etiology of hydrothorax is not always determined, and idiopathic pleural effusion is frustrating and challenging to treat.

Hemothorax

Pathophysiology

Accumulation of blood in the pleural space occurs because of trauma, a systemic coagulopathy, lung lobe torsion, or neoplasia. A coagulation defect associated with clotting factor deficiency or inhibition due to rodenticide intoxication is more likely to result in hemorrhage into a body cavity than is a defect in platelet numbers or function.

History and signalment

Young animals are more likely to suffer trauma or develop a coagulopathy secondary to rodenticide intoxication while older animals are more likely to develop a hemorrhagic effusion due to neoplasia. Lung lobe torsion is reported in any age animal. Systemic signs of weakness and blood loss may predominate over respiratory abnormalities. Rodenticide intoxication generally results in clinical signs 2–5 days postingestion and signs of weakness and respiratory difficulty are often acute in onset. Dogs with neoplasia or lung lobe torsion may have a gradual onset of lethargy or weakness followed by difficult or rapid breathing.

Physical examination

Animals with a coagulopathy can demonstrate pale mucous membranes, tachycardia, or evidence of hemorrhage elsewhere in the body, such as the abdominal cavity, skin (ecchymotic hemorrhages), joints, or eyes (hyphema or retinal bleeding). Tachypnea is often evident when pleural fluid is present, and heart and lung sounds will be muffled. Increased or harsh lung sounds may be auscultated focally when parenchymal neoplasia is present.

Diagnostic findings

Radiographs reveal pleural effusion and in animals with a coagulopathy, parenchymal and mediastinal infiltrates are usually found that are more severe than the pleural effusion (Berry et al. 2005). Bony structures of the thorax should be scrutinized for rib fractures in suspected trauma patients. Radiographs or ultrasound can be useful in detecting pulmonary lesions such as neoplasia or lung lobe torsion (see Chapter 6) that might lead to hemothorax.

In an animal with hemothorax due to pure hemorrhage or a coagulopathy, the packed cell volume (PCV) of the pleural fluid will approach that of the systemic PCV. Additional evidence of hemorrhage can be found in laboratory results including anemia, mild to moderate thrombocytopenia, and hypoalbuminemia. Prolongation of tests for secondary hemostasis confirms a coagulopathy (Figure 7.9). The one-stage prothrombin time (OSPT) provides an assessment of the extrinsic coagulation pathway and vitamin K-dependent factors while the activated partial thromboplastin time (APTT) evaluates the intrinsic and common pathway.

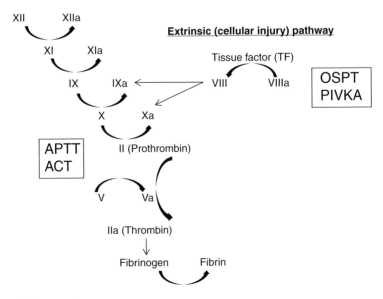

Figure 7.9. Coagulation cascade.

In an emergency room, the activated clotting time (ACT) is often used to assess the intrinsic and common pathway. Controversy exists regarding the use of the PIVKA test (proteins induced by vitamin K antagonists) for differentiating anticoagulant poisoning from other causes of coagulopathy because the test is similar to the OSPT, although dramatic prolongation (>150 seconds) appears suggestive of intoxication (Mount et al. 2003).

Treatment

If a coagulopathy is documented, it is usually not necessary or wise to drain the chest because respiratory distress in these patients is often due to parenchymal bleeding rather than pleural accumulation of blood. For rapid reestablishment of clotting ability, fresh frozen plasma should be administered at 6–10 mL/kg initially. Fresh whole blood transfusion is indicated if the animal is anemic. Vitamin K_1 is initiated concurrently at a loading dose of 5 mg/kg SC (using a small gauge needle) followed by 1.5–2.5 mg/kg PO twice daily for 21–30 days. Clotting times are reassessed during the initial 1–3 days of stabilization period and again 2–3 days after halting therapy.

Conservative management of hemothorax due to trauma is warranted initially with oxygen supplementation and judicious use of pain relief and sedation. Surgical intervention could be required if an artery is severed or if a broken rib causes persistent bleeding.

Prognosis

Animals that are documented to have a coagulopathy usually respond well to vitamin K therapy, although it is important to obtain follow-up testing to ensure normalization of clotting tests after the drug is discontinued.

Feline Infectious Peritonitis (Coronavirus)

Pathophysiology

The disease syndrome associated with feline infectious peritonitis (FIP) is initiated when an enteric coronavirus undergoes spontaneous mutation into a virulent form that triggers immune-mediated disease. It appears that a strong cell-mediated immune response protects against the virus while the humoral response may promote immunologically driven disease. The clinical syndrome associated with FIP is characterized by two forms of disease. The effusive or wet form is thought to be associated with a strong humoral response that leads to an immune complex vasculitis with increased vascular permeability and neutrophil-mediated vessel necrosis. Pleural, peritoneal, and pericardial effusions develop. The noneffusive disease or dry form is thought to result from an ineffectual cell-mediated response by the host to contain the virus. Pyogranulomatous inflammation accompanied by vasculitis develops in any organ, including liver, kidney, lung, or brain. Some evidence suggests that there can be a transition between effusive and noneffusive disease.

History and signalment

Mutation of the coronavirus and subsequent FIP-related disease are more common in young animals from multicat households, suggesting that environmental stresses play a role in the etiopathogenesis of disease. FIP most commonly affects purebred kittens and young cats 2–16 months of age, but it can occur in any age of cat. Owner complaints include a failure to thrive, anorexia, and weight loss. Progressive abdominal enlargement is often noted over weeks to months and may be accompanied by respiratory difficulty. Tachypnea and respiratory distress may be noted because of the presence of granulomatous pneumonia or pleural effusion.

Physical examination

Cats with FIP usually have a fever and, in the effusive form, will display signs of abdominal and/or thoracic effusion. Abdominal distention, a ballotable fluid wave, muffled heart and lung sounds, and tachypnea are common features in affected cats.

Organ involvement by the dry form of FIP can result in chorioretinitis, neurologic deficits, irregular contours to the liver or kidneys, or diffuse or focal thickening of intestines. Granulomatous pneumonia results in tachypnea and harsh lung sounds.

Diagnostic findings

Clinical diagnosis of FIP is often suspected based on the presence of fever and thoracic and/or abdominal effusion in a young cat. Laboratory findings consistent with a diagnosis include anemia, lymphopenia, neutrophilia, hyperglobulinemia with a polyclonal gammopathy, and decreased serum albumin/globulin ratio (<0.6). A very high coronavirus titer ($>1:1600$) is supportive of disease and a negative titer makes FIP less likely; however, antibody titers are not specific for the mutated virus. Abdominal or thoracic fluid is generally yellow, viscous and highly proteinaceous (proteins 4–10 g/dL) with variable cellularity (2000–25,000 cells/μL). Immunocytochemistry for detection of viral antigen in effusion is currently the most useful noninvasive diagnostic test for FIP (Hartmann et al. 2003).

Real-time reverse-transcriptase PCR on pleural or peritoneal fluid that yields a positive result for feline coronavirus is suggestive of FIP-related disease since the virus should not be detected outside the gastrointestinal tract. However the test confirms only the presence of coronavirus, not the presence of the mutated virulent form responsible for disease. Definitive diagnosis requires invasive testing to identify characteristic histopathologic lesions of pyogranulomatous inflammation and necrotizing vasculitis. Immunohistochemistry for viral antigens confirms the diagnosis.

Treatment

No specific antiviral treatment has been developed for FIP-related disease. Interferon-omega therapy had no effect on survival time in one study (Ritz et al. 2007). Supportive care with intravenous fluid therapy, nutritional support, and repeated fluid drainage can be used to keep the cat comfortable.

Prognosis

FIP is fatal within days to months in virtually every case. Control of the disease in populations relies on management strategies that limit crowding, stress, and other illnesses in the environment. Genetic resistance or susceptibility in breeding lines should be evaluated to help control disease within populations.

Chylothorax

Pathophysiology

Chylothorax is caused by leakage of lymphatic fluid from the thoracic duct into the pleural cavity. It is seen in both dogs and cats. The etiology is often idiopathic; however, diseases associated with increased right heart pressures, such as cardiomyopathy, pericardial disease, congenital heart disease, and heartworm disease, have been reported as potential causes. Mediastinal masses (lymphosarcoma, thymoma) have been diagnosed in association with chylothorax, and chylothorax is seen in dogs with lung lobe torsion. Traumatic rupture of the thoracic duct is a relatively rare cause of chylothorax

History and signalment

Afghan hounds are thought to be predisposed to development of chylothorax and are a breed that is susceptible to lung lobe torsion, although the relationship between these two disorders remains unclear.

Clinical signs of pleural disease (respiratory abnormalities) may be acute or chronic. In one study, a relatively high percentage of cats (30%) had a history of cough as well as labored breathing. This is likely due to airway compression from restricted lung expansion. Some animals may suffer weight loss associated with loss of protein, fat, and vitamins into lymph fluid in the chest.

Physical examination

Some animals may have a poor body condition score. Tachypnea and/or labored respirations are expected when fluid fills the pleural space. Heart and lung sounds are muffled ventrally or unilaterally (because chyle can plug mediastinal fenestrae). Harsh or adventitious lung sounds are common. Careful cardiac auscultation should be performed to detect a murmur, gallop, or arrhythmia that might suggest heart disease as an underlying cause of chylous effusion.

Diagnostic findings

Radiographic or physical examination evidence of pleural effusion indicates that thoracocentesis should be performed. In chylothorax, unilateral or bilateral effusion may be present, and a characteristic white or pink opaque fluid is obtained on chest tap (Figure 7.10). Chylothorax is diagnosed by performing cholesterol and triglyceride analysis on pleural fluid and serum. Because chyle is lymphatic fluid, triglyceride levels in pleural fluid are significantly higher than in serum, and cholesterol levels are lower than in serum. A cholesterol/triglyceride ratio <0.2 in pleural fluid is considered diagnostic for chylothorax. Once the diagnosis of chylothorax has been established, further diagnostic tests are performed

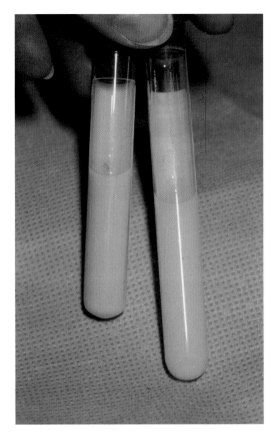

Figure 7.10. Chylous effusion is typically opaque due to the presence of chylomicrons and may be white or pink, depending on whether blood contamination has occurred.

to determine whether an underlying cause can be identified. Such tests include pleural fluid cytology, heartworm testing, echocardiography, thoracic ultrasound, and abdominal ultrasound.

Treatment

Initial therapy for chylothorax should be directed at the cause when identified. Thoracocentesis should be performed whenever the animal develops respiratory difficulty. Dietary therapy with reduced fat and supplementation with medium chain triglyceride oil has historically been the mainstay of treatment because it was thought that these changes would reduce lymph flow. Some animals may benefit from this therapy but clinical studies have not confirmed that they will substantially decrease lymph flow. Adjunctive dietary therapy with rutin, a benzopyrone, at 50 mg/kg PO TID has had moderate success in reducing chyle accumulation in some patients, and relatively few side effects have been reported. The mechanism of action is unknown, but this agent may stimulate macrophages to remove

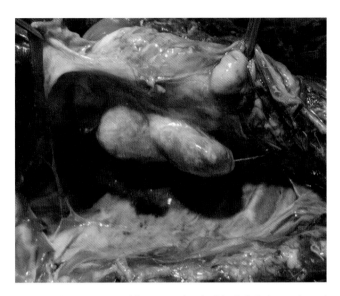

Figure 7.11. Necropsy image from a 5 year old FS DSH that had had chylothorax for at least 2–3 months. The lungs did not collapse after the chest was opened, and fibrin was evident between the right lung lobes and visceral pleura. Both the parietal and visceral pleura were markedly thickened.

lymph protein, decrease leakage of fluid from blood vessels, or enhance proteolysis and removal of protein from tissues.

When thoracocentesis is required more often than once per week, surgical options should be considered. Surgical therapy with thoracic duct ligation and pericardiectomy has recently been reported as 80–100% effective as therapy for chylothorax in dogs and cats (Fossum et al. 2004). CT-guided injection of the mesenteric lymph node improves visualization of the thoracic duct and avoids the need for an abdominal surgery (Johnson et al. 2009).

Prognosis

Fibrosing pleuritis is a debilitating condition that can occur after long-standing high-protein pleural effusion, such as chylothorax or pyothorax. Chronic inflammation of the pleura results in metaplasia of mesothelial cells with production of collagen, and the presence of pleural fluid decreases fibrinolysis resulting in an increased collagen network within the pleura. Thickened pleura restricts lung expansion (Figure 7.11). Pleural effusion may or may not be present in later stages of disease. The radiographic appearance of fibrosing pleuritis is characterized by persistently unexpanded and rounded lung lobe margins (Figure 7.12).

Therapy for fibrosing pleuritis involves surgical decortication of the pleura. This procedure has been beneficial in humans if less than two lobes are affected; however, most affected animals have generalized pleuritis, which is not easily treated with surgery. Complications of the surgery include pneumothorax and hemorrhage. If surgery is performed, steroids should be considered for 2–3 weeks postoperatively. Lung function may improve over 2–3 months.

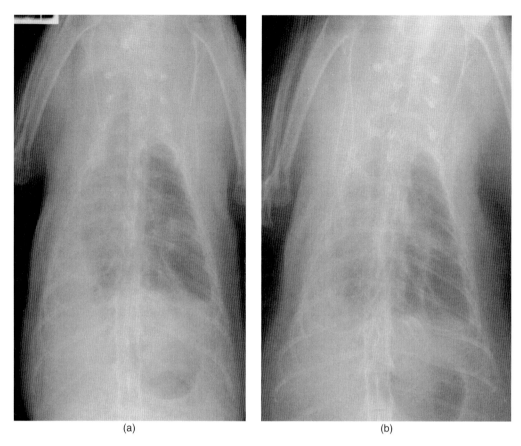

(a)   (b)

Figure 7.12.   Dorsoventral radiographs from a cat pre- (a) and post- (b) thoracocentesis. Note that the lung margins are rounded and remain unexpanded despite removal of pleural fluid. Necropsy revealed fibrosing pleuritis.

References

Au JJ, Weisman DL, Stefanacci JD, Palmisano MP. Use of computed tomography for evaluation of lung lesions associated with spontaneous pneumothorax in dogs: 12 cases (1999–2002). J Am Vet Med Assoc. 2006; 228: 733–737.

Berry CR, Gallawy A, Thrall DE, Carlisle C. Thoracic radiographic features of anticoagulant rodenticide toxicity in fourteen dogs. Vet Rad Ultrasound. 2005; 34: 391–396.

Bowman DD, Frongillo MK, Johnson RC, et al. Evaluation of praziquantel for treatment of experimentally induced paragonimiasis in dogs and cats. Am J Vet Res. 1991; 52: 68–71.

Dvir E, Kirberger RM, Malleczek D. Radiographic and computed tomographic changes and clinical presentation of spirocercosis in the dog. Vet Radiol Ultrasound. 2001; 42: 119–129.

Fossum TW, Mertens MM, Miller MW, et al. Thoracic duct ligation and pericardectomy for treatment of idiopathic chylothorax. J Vet Int Med. 2004; 18: 307–310.

Gibson TWG, Brisson BA, Sears W. Perioperative survival rates after surgery for diaphragmatic hernia in dogs and cats: 92 cases (1990–2002). J Am Vet Med Assoc. 2005: 227; 105–109.

Hartmann K, Binder C, Hirschberger J, et al. Comparison of different tests to diagnose feline infectious peritonitis. J Vet Int Med. 2003; 17: 781–790.

Johnson EG, Wisner ER, Kyles A, et al. Computed tomographic lymphography of the thoracic duct by mesenteric lymph node injection. Vet Surg. 2009; 38: 361–367.

Johnson MS, Martin MWS. Successful medical treatment of 15 dogs with pyothorax. J Small Anim Pract. 2007; 48: 12–16.

Lana S, Plaza S, Hampe K, et al. Diagnosis of mediastinal masses in dogs by flow cytometry. J Vet Int Med. 2006; 20: 1161–1165.

Louwerens M, London CA, Pedersen NC, Lyons LA. Feline lymphoma in the post-feline leukemia virus era. J Vet Int Med. 2005; 19: 329–335.

Mount ME, Kim BU, Kass PH. Use of a test for proteins induced by vitamin K absence or antagonism in diagnosis of anticoagulant poisoning in dogs: 325 cases (1987–1997). J Am Vet Med Assoc. 2003; 222: 194–198.

Puerto DA, Brockman DJ, Lindquist C, Drobatz K. Surgical and nonsurgical management of selected risk factors for spontaneous pneumothorax in dogs: 64 cases (1986–1999). J Am Vet Med Assoc. 2002: 220; 1670–1674.

Ritz S, Egberink H, Hartmann K. Effect of feline interferon-omega on the survival time and quality of life of cats with feline infectious peritonitis. J Vet Int Med. 2007; 21: 1193–1197.

Teske E, van Straten G, van Noort R, Rutteman GR. Chemotherapy with cyclophosphamide, vincristine, and prednisolone (COP) in cats with malignant lymphoma: new results with an old protocol. J Vet Int Med. 2002; 16: 179–186.

Walker AL, Jang SS, Hirsch DC. Bacteria associated with pyothorax in dogs and cats: 98 cases (1989–1998). J Am Vet Med Assoc. 2000; 216: 359–363.

Vascular Disorders 8

Structural Disorders

Pulmonary Thromboembolism

Pathophysiology

Systemic diseases that result in stasis of blood flow, hypercoagulability, and disruption of the endothelial layer of the vascular bed can result in the secondary complication of pulmonary thromboembolism (PTE). In dogs, immune-mediated hemolytic anemia, sepsis, neoplasia, amyloidosis, hyperadrenocorticism, and dilated cardiomyopathy are associated with increased risk for PTE, while neoplasia and cardiomyopathy are found most often in cats with PTE (Johnson et al. 1999b, Norris et al. 1999)

PTE results in multiple pathophysiologic events that affect gas exchange. Physical obstruction of large pulmonary arteries by clot material increases intravascular pressure, and release of clot-associated vasoactive factors (e.g., thromboxane) causes reactive pulmonary vasoconstriction. Elaboration of humoral mediators (e.g., serotonin, histamine, calcium, and growth factors) from platelets results in bronchoconstriction and increased airway resistance. Surfactant function is altered leading to loss of elastic recoil and atelectasis, decreased pulmonary compliance, and increased right-to-left shunting. Alveolar dead space is increased because of the presence of nonperfused lung regions, and this leads to increased work of breathing.

History and signalment

PTE is generally a disorder of older animals, and history and clinical signs reflect the underlying disease process. Acute onset of respiratory distress and tachypnea in any seriously ill animal should trigger suspicion for PTE. Recent trauma or surgery might also lead to PTE.

Physical examination

Animals with PTE often display relentless tachypnea and breathlessness that is refractory to supplemental oxygen administration. Harsh lung sounds or loud bronchovesicular sounds can be detected; however, crackles or wheezes are less common. Physical examination abnormalities usually reflect the underlying disease process. For example, pale mucous membranes are present in animals with immune-mediated hemolytic anemia, a heart murmur or gallop in the patient with cardiac disease, or a pot-bellied appearance in the dog with Cushing's disease.

Diagnostic findings

Diagnostic testing is directed at determining the underlying cause for embolization and assessing the severity of gas exchange abnormalities. Thoracic radiographs can be relatively unremarkable (Figure 8.1); however, a variety of pulmonary infiltrates have been reported

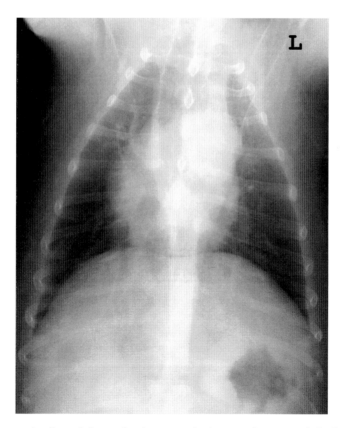

Figure 8.1.   Dorsoventral radiograph from a dog documented to have a pulmonary embolus in the lobar artery to the right caudal lung lobe. Note the lack of pulmonary infiltrates, pleural effusion, or vascular abnormalities.

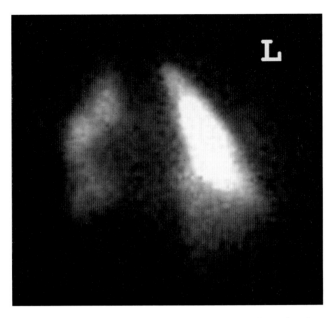

Figure 8.2. Perfusion scan from the dog depicted in Figure 8.1 indicates a lack of perfusion in the right caudal lung lobe, consistent with major pulmonary embolus affecting the blood supply to that lung lobe.

in dogs with PTE. Cats may be more likely to exhibit pulmonary vascular abnormalities such as uneven distribution of perfusion or blunted pulmonary vessels (Norris et al. 1999), and this might facilitate early diagnosis of PTE. A coagulation panel is generally indicated in the work-up of suspected PTE to assess the intrinsic pathway (APTT, ACT), the extrinsic pathway (OSPT), and fibrin degradation products (FDPs) or D-dimer (see Figure 7.9). Unfortunately, assay for D-dimer, a breakdown product of cross-linked fibrin, has not proven sensitive or specific in documentation of PTE. Thromboelastography, a technique that can identify hypo- and hypercoagulable states by assessing the speed, efficiency, and strength of clot formation, may prove useful in both the diagnosis and management of patients at risk for PTE.

Confirmation of embolization is difficult and requires perfusion scanning with 99-technetium-labeled macroaggregated albumin (Figure 8.2), ventilation/perfusion scanning, or computed tomography (CT) angiography. Perfusion scanning can be a valuable clinical tool because it can be done in the awake animal. This technique has documented that pulmonary embolization is common in dogs after cemented total hip replacement (Liska and Poteet 2003); however, this technique has not been evaluated for use in patients with cardiopulmonary disease and other risk factors for PTE because of the need for anesthesia to complete the scan. Echocardiography might be helpful in increasing suspicion for the diagnosis, since a clot may be visible in the right atrium, or indirect evidence of right ventricular overload might be seen such as right ventricular dilation, flattening of the right ventricular septum, or pulmonary hypertension.

Treatment

Control of the primary disease process is essential in managing PTE. Oxygen therapy is recommended for animals with PTE, although the respiratory pattern may not improve dramatically because of alterations in central respiratory control. Animals that do not have intrapulmonary shunting will show improved hemoglobin saturation with oxygen while on supplementation; however, not all dogs with PTE are oxygen responsive (Johnson et al. 1999b).

Medical therapy for both treatment and prevention of PTE is aimed at limiting further deposition of fibrin on existing clots. Heparin bound to antithrombin inactivates factors (thrombin factor (IIa), factors Xa, IXa, XIa, and XIIa) and prevents further accumulation of fibrin on a clot. Subcutaneous heparin (200–300 U/kg SQ BID–TID) is administered to prolong the APTT two to three times the normal value. In most hospitals, the use of heparin has been supplanted by low-molecular-weight heparins (LMWH). Examples of LMWH agents include enoxaparin (Lovenox®) and dalteparin (Fragmin®). This class of drug acts similarly to heparin in inhibiting further clot formation but has greater inhibition of factor X versus factor II, and therefore does not prolong the APTT. Experimental studies in dogs have revealed improved antithrombotic efficacy of LMWH over unfractionated heparin. In cats, LMWH given at standard doses (enoxaparin at 1 mg/kg SQ BID) resulted in plasma levels that approach the human therapeutic range 4 hours after dosing, while administration of dalteparin (100 IU/kg BID) resulted in less predictable levels (Alwood et al. 2007, Vargo et al. 2009). Also, enoxaparin was rapidly cleared, suggesting that more frequent administration may be required.

Antiplatelet therapy may also reduce the risk of clotting. A low dose of aspirin is used to inhibit cyclooxygenase activity without reducing endothelial cell production of prostacyclin. Although the precise dosage is not certain in veterinary species, 1–2 mg/kg/day in the dog appears to limit platelet aggregation. It is difficult to achieve this small dose in the cat, and because of its prolonged half-life, aspirin is dosed every 2–3 days. Aspirin therapy can be used concurrently with other drugs to decrease platelet aggregability. A newer class of drugs (thienopyridine class) being used to inhibit platelet function acts at the glycoprotein IIb/IIIa receptor and decreases aggregation as well as fibrin cross-linkage. One such drug, clopidogrel (Plavix®), has been shown to be safe and effective at inhibiting platelets in *healthy* cats at dosages of 18.75 to 75 mg once daily (Hogan et al. 2004), and various experimental studies in dogs (2–4 mg/kg/day) have shown that it reduces clotting. Use of these drugs in clinical disease is under investigation.

With increasing certainty of the diagnosis of PTE or worsening condition of the patient, more aggressive therapy with fibrinolytic agents can be considered (tissue plasminogen activator, streptokinase). The efficacy of this therapy has not been established in animals with PTE, and in human medicine, fibrinolytic therapy is reserved for patients with hemodynamic instability.

Prognosis

Development of PTE is associated with a guarded prognosis, and mortality is high. Because of the poor success in treatment of PTE, prophylactic anticoagulant therapy should be considered in animals with diseases that have been shown to predispose to the condition. Low-dose aspirin is advised for platelet inhibition. Various doses of heparin have been recommended for prophylaxis: 10 U/kg SQ TID (mini-dose regimen) or 60–100 U/kg SQ BID–TID (low-dose regimen). These dosages should not prolong APTT. LMWH are more costly but can also be used as prophylaxis against embolization. Monitoring thromboelastography and performing an antifactor Xa assay (Cornell University) can be used to determine the dose that approximates the known therapeutic range in humans.

Infectious Disorders

Canine Heartworm Disease

Pathophysiology

Canine heartworm disease is a condition with essentially worldwide distribution dependent on the presence of the mosquito vector. It is most common in warm, humid environments with highest infection rates along the east coast of the United States, Gulf States, and Mississippi river valley. Mosquitoes deposit third-stage larvae of *Dirofilaria immitis* under the skin. The larvae migrate into the right heart and pulmonary arterial system where they develop into adult worms and begin producing microfilaria 5–7 months after infection. High worm burden is common in infected dogs, and disease results from obstruction of pulmonary arteries followed by right ventricular failure due to pressure overload. Heartworms also trigger pulmonary endothelial damage that can stimulate clot formation with subsequent thromboembolization. Physical damage to the adult worm or death of the adult can result in worm embolization. Heartworms also trigger a pulmonary hypersensitivity response that results in eosinophilic inflammation in the parenchyma. Antigen–antibody complex deposition in the kidneys can lead to a protein losing glomerulonephritis, and heartworm infection can also cause hepatocellular damage.

History and signalment

Heartworm disease can be detected in dogs with no clinical complaints, or owners may note coughing, exercise intolerance, or an abnormal breathing pattern. Dogs with severe infections develop hemoptysis and signs of right-sided heart failure, pulmonary hypertension, or pulmonary thromboembolization pulmonary embolization including respiratory distress, abdominal distension, and syncope.

Physical examination

Dogs may lack any physical manifestations of heartworm disease. In dogs with mild disease, tracheal sensitivity may be present. With progressive severity of infection, dogs may appear cachectic and display manifestations of right-sided heart failure, including ascites or hepatomegaly, icterus, jugular venous distension, a heart murmur or gallop rhythm, loss of lung sounds due to pleural effusion or crackles associated with parenchymal disease.

Diagnostic findings

Peripheral eosinophilia is commonly detected on a complete blood count in infected dogs. Chemistry panel and urinalysis should be closely scrutinized for evidence of liver dysfunction (indicated by an increase in alanine transaminase) and renal involvement (indicated by elevated blood urea nitrogen, increased creatinine, or the presence of proteinuria). When proteinuria is detected, a urine protein-to-creatinine ratio is recommended to gain an appreciation of the severity of glomerulonephritis.

Microfilaria can be detected by a modified Knott's or filter test; however, microfilaremia will be found only in infected dogs that are not on heartworm-preventive medication.

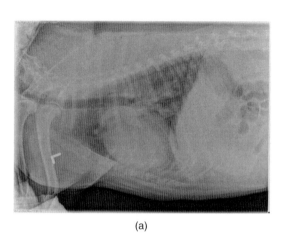
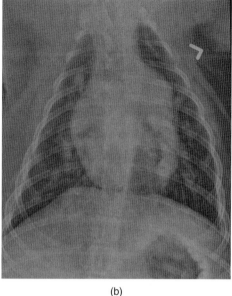

(a)   (b)

Figure 8.3.   Left lateral (a) and dorsoventral (b) radiographs from an 8-year-old FS Shepherd mix dog with stage 3 heartworm disease. There is severe enlargement of pulmonary arteries, with a bulge at the region of the main pulmonary artery on the dorsoventral projection and rounding of the cranial aspect of the heart on the lateral projection consistent with right-sided cardiomegaly. Diffuse pulmonary infiltrates are noted along with mild enlargement of the caudal vena cava and liver. (Courtesy of Dr. Adonia Hsu, University of California, Davis.)

Therefore, because most dogs are on some form of preventive, an antigen test is the recommended screening test. The test will be positive 6–7 months after infection, although a false-negative antigen test can be encountered with infection by immature worms or all males. When a positive antigen test is obtained, blood should be assessed for microfilaria.

Radiographic findings in canine heartworm disease vary depending on the severity of disease. Pulmonary arteries become progressively enlarged, blunted, and tortuous, parenchymal infiltrates progress, and right ventricular enlargement develops (Figure 8.3). Echocardiography detects the walls of the heartworm as parallel lines (Figure 8.4) and can demonstrate signs of right ventricular overload including right ventricular dilatation, tricuspid regurgitation, and pulmonary hypertension.

Treatment

Prior to adulticidal treatment, the severity of disease should be staged and clinical signs stabilized as indicated. In addition, owners should be cautioned about the possibility of embolic disease and should understand the need for cage confinement for 1–2 months to limit the occurrence of this complication. Monthly preventive medication is continued in dogs with occult infection. If microfilaria are present, the initial dose of preventive medication should be given to the dog while hospitalized to monitor for adverse effects.

Melarsomine dihydrochloride is the approved adulticidal treatment of canine heartworm disease. The manufacturer provides the following recommendations for treatment based on the severity of disease (although the American Heartworm Society and many clinicians

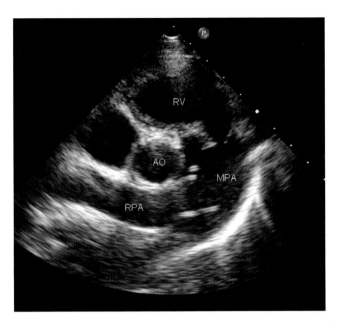

Figure 8.4. Echocardiographic image from the dog depicted in Figure 8.3 demonstrates parallel lines in the right pulmonary artery (RPA) characteristic of heartworm infection. AO, aorta; RV, right ventricle; MPA, main pulmonary artery (Courtesy of Dr. Adonia Hsu, University of California, Davis.)

prefer to treat all dogs with the split dose protocol). Class 1 dogs are mildly affected with few clinical signs and normal radiographs and laboratory findings. Class 2 dogs are moderately affected with cough or respiratory difficulty, have right heart enlargement on radiographs, and have abnormal laboratory values such as anemia or elevated liver enzymes. Dogs in these groups are given two deep intramuscular injections of melarsomine (2.5 mg/kg) between the third and fifth lumbar vertebrae on alternate sides of the spine separated by 24 hours. Dogs are kept confined and monitored by respiratory rate and effort for adverse effects. For dogs with persistent clinical signs and positive antigen test, a second treatment can be given in 4 months. Class 3 dogs are severely affected with signs of right heart failure, severe radiographic abnormalities, and marked laboratory abnormalities. These dogs appear to be at higher risk for embolization and should be stabilized prior to treatment with oxygen, diuretics, and angiotensin-converting enzyme inhibitors. Use of anticoagulants is controversial. In these dogs, the split-dose protocol is recommended by using a single deep intramuscular injection of melarsomine followed one month later by two injections given 24 hours apart. Restriction of physical activity is essential for 4–6 weeks after treatment. Class 4 dogs are those with caval syndrome, and melarsomine is not recommended for these dogs. Stabilization and physical removal of worms are required.

Any circulating microfilaria or developing larvae are eliminated over 6–9 months through administration of heartworm preventive medications. Ivermectin and milbemycin oxime are oral preparations given monthly. Milbemycin is preferred for collies or any collie-type dogs that might have the deletion mutation of the *mdr1* (multidrug-resistance-1) gene. Selamectin and moxidectin are topically administered drugs that prevent heartworm disease. Moxidectin is also available as an injectable product that provides 6 months of prevention.

Prognosis

Dogs with mild-to-moderate heartworm disease have a good prognosis for uneventful treatment and full recovery, although melarsomine can be associated with various toxicities, including injection site reaction and neurologic signs (Hettlich et al. 2003). Dogs with Class 3 and 4 diseases are at increased risk for embolization during and after treatment, and may develop long-term pulmonary disease associated with pulmonary arterial damage.

Feline Heartworm Disease

Pathophysiology

The initial life cycle of heartworm in the cat is similar to that in the dog, with deposition of L3 larvae under the skin followed by development into adult worms in the pulmonary artery approximately 3–4 months after infection. However, in the cat, infection with only one to six adult worms is typical and single sex infection is common. This feature, along with an augmented host response to the microfilaria, may explain the lack of microfilaremia in most cats. Interestingly, aberrant migration of heartworm larvae is relatively common in the cat, and cerebral infection is a potential cause for sudden death in cats. Antibody production can be detected within 2–3 months of infection, and heartworm antigen is present from 5.5 to 8 months postinfection.

Signs of pulmonary disease may arise from infection with adult heartworms or the effect of larval stages on lung vasculature (Browne et al. 2005). Sudden death may result from an anaphylactic response to internal filarial antigens released with worm death (Litster et al. 2008).

History and signalment

Both indoor and outdoor cats can be infected with heartworm through mosquito exposure. Young to middle-aged cats are affected most commonly but cats of any age can be infected. Many cats do not develop disease associated with heartworm, but it has been recognized as a cause of a multitude of clinical signs including chronic cough, acute respiratory distress, vomiting unrelated to eating, neurologic signs, and lethargy. Sudden death is a relatively common occurrence, and in some cats, respiratory or gastrointestinal signs are noted immediately before death.

Physical examination

There are no specific physical examination findings indicative of feline heartworm disease. Cats may display tracheal sensitivity or adventitious lung sounds associated with pulmonary disease.

Diagnostic findings

Diagnosis of feline heartworm disease can be difficult. Peripheral eosinophilia is present in <50% of cases. Radiographic changes that characterize feline heartworm disease are reflected by enlargement of caudal pulmonary lobar arteries (Figure 8.5), although in one study of naturally infected cats, abnormalities in pulmonary vasculature were uncommon

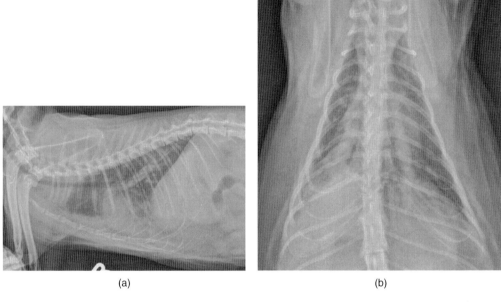

(a)   (b)

Figure 8.5. Right lateral (a) and dorsoventral (b) radiographs from a 4-year-old FS Himalayan mix with severe heartworm disease reveal moderate, generalized cardiac enlargement characterized by rounding of the caudal cardiac silhouette. The main pulmonary artery is enlarged and there is severe enlargement and blunting of caudal lobar pulmonary arteries. Diffuse peribronchial infiltrates and mild pleural effusion are also present. (Courtesy of Dr. Mike Cocchiaro, University of California, Davis.)

(Venco et al. 2008). Unlike dogs, cardiac chambers are unlikely to be changed by heartworm infection. Focal or diffuse bronchointerstitial infiltrates are the most common parenchymal changes in cats with heartworm but presence of infiltrates depends on the stage of disease (Venco et al. 2008).

Heartworm antibody positivity indicates only exposure to heartworm, and false-negative tests are unfortunately common. The antigen test can detect a single female heartworm but may be falsely negative when no females are present or only a few live males are present. Heartworm disease can be diagnosed on echocardiography by the presence of two parallel hyperechoic lines in the right ventricle or pulmonary artery.

Treatment

Treatment of feline heartworm disease is based on control of clinical signs. In an acute presentation, intravenous corticosteroids, terbutaline, and oxygen therapy should be provided. In more chronic cases, the pulmonary hypersensitivity response is treated with a tapering dose of prednisolone as required while waiting for the heartworms to die (generally within 3–4 years). Use of aspirin is controversial as its role in preventing embolic disease is uncertain, and it should not be administered concurrently with steroids.

Adulticidal therapy is not currently recommended because melarsomine has not been fully evaluated in the cat. For cats with severe signs associated with pulmonary artery obstruction, physical removal of worms from the heart through jugular venotomy and use of intravenous snares or baskets can be performed when the worms are accessible. Caution is warranted to prevent breakage of the worm during removal and possible anaphylaxis.

Radiographs and serology should be repeated every 6–12 months as needed until pulmonary lesions have resolved and the antigen test is negative.

Prognosis

Many cats appear to tolerate infection with heartworm without development of clinical signs and the immune system will clear the infection over several years. Some cats develop severe refractory clinical signs, and feline heartworm disease can cause sudden death in 20–30% of cats with clinical signs. For cats at risk, monthly ivermectin (24 µg/kg PO), milbemycin oxime (2 mg/kg PO), selamectin (6–12 mg/kg topically), or 10% imidacloprid/1% moxidectin (applied topically) given year round afford protection against feline heartworm disease. Preventive treatment may also reduce worm burden in cats that are already infected. Updated guidelines on feline heartworm disease are available from the American Heartworm Society.

French Heartworm Disease

Pathophysiology

Vascular infection with the metastrongyloid worm *Angiostrongylus vasorum* is responsible for the disease known as French heartworm disease. The worm is endemic in certain parts of the United Kingdom, Europe, and South America and has spread to Newfoundland, Canada (Chapman et al. 2004, Bourque et al. 2008). This worm infects dogs and foxes as its definitive host and is spread through ingestion of intermediate or paratenic hosts, including slugs, snails, and frogs. Disease is initiated by ingestion of the intermediate host containing infective third-stage larvae. Larvae are released in the dog's intestine, gain access to the circulation, and migrate to the pulmonary artery, right heart, and pulmonary arterioles where development into the adult stage is completed. The prepatent period is 40–60 days. Eggs travel to the pulmonary capillaries where first-stage larvae hatch and migrate into the alveolus where they are coughed up, swallowed, and passed in the feces to be taken up by the intermediate host. Maturation into infective L3 occurs in the intermediate host.

Respiratory disease results from the inflammatory response induced by migration of the larvae, which causes granulomatous pneumonia and thrombotic disease (Bourque et al. 2008). Right heart failure appears to be less common than that seen with *Dirofilaria immitis*, perhaps because of the smaller size of *Angiostrongylus* (1.5–2 cm). A hemorrhagic diathesis has also been reported with *Angiostrongylus* infection. The precise mechanism is unclear but may be related to a consumptive coagulopathy.

History and signalment

Outdoor dogs and those that hunt are exposed to possible infection more commonly than other dogs; however, both urban and rural dogs can be affected (Chapman et al. 2004). Infection seems more common in younger dogs, and dogs are presented for a combination of signs including coughing, exercise intolerance, respiratory distress, evidence of hemorrhage (ecchymotic hemorrhages, hemoptysis, gingival bleeding), and/or syncope.

Physical examination

Dogs with a bleeding diathesis will display ecchymotic hemorrhage in the subcutis, conjunctiva, sclera, or mucous membranes. Overt bleeding from mucosal surfaces may be present. Pneumonia results in tachypnea and respiratory difficulty. Abnormal or harsh lung sounds may be auscultated.

Diagnostic findings

Eosinophilia or neutrophilia can be seen on a complete blood count, and hyperglobulinemia is relatively common (Chapman et al. 2004). A platelet count should be assessed in dogs suspected of angiostrongylosis because thrombocytopenia is common. A coagulation panel (OSPT, APTT) is recommended given the possibility for infection to result in a coagulopathy. Thoracic radiographs generally show an interstitial to alveolar pattern that is concentrated in the caudodorsal lung fields, reflecting the pulmonary hypersensitivity response to larval migration.

Infection with this helminth is best confirmed through the use of a fecal Baermann analysis for L1 stages. Bronchoalveolar lavage can detect the first-stage larvae and will provide information on the type and severity of the pulmonary inflammation. No information is available on the utility of a tracheal wash specimen for detecting larvae.

Treatment

Successful treatment of infection has been reported with a single dose of 0.1 mL/kg bodyweight of imidacloprid 10%/moxidectin 2.5% spot-on solution or with fenbendazole (25–50 mg/kg PO for 20 days) (Chapman 2004, Willesen et al. 2007). Depending on the severity of clinical signs and pulmonary infiltrates, additional therapy with corticosteroids, intravenous fluid support, and oxygen can be required.

Prognosis

Dogs with low worm burdens may remain subclinical. Animals with severe radiographic changes, marked respiratory difficulty, or syncope have a guarded prognosis for recovery. It appears that dogs surviving to discharge experience few residual effects of disease.

Miscellaneous Disorders

Pulmonary Hypertension

Pathophysiology

Pulmonary hypertension (PH) can complicate a variety of congenital or acquired cardiac and pulmonary conditions. Classifications of PH include pulmonary arterial hypertension (usually of idiopathic origin), pulmonary venous hypertension associated with increased left atrial pressure, PH associated with thrombosis, PH associated with respiratory disease, and miscellaneous causes of PH. Idiopathic pulmonary arteriopathy resulting in PH has been reported rarely in the veterinary literature (Glaus et al. 2004, Zabka et al. 2006). Pulmonary venous hypertension associated with left heart disease is relatively common although the elevation in PA pressure is often mild to moderate. PH associated with respiratory disease results from increased vascular resistance due to primary or secondary obstructive or obliterative diseases of the vasculature or from chronic and global hypoxic vasoconstriction. In veterinary medicine, the most well-recognized cause of pulmonary hypertension is heartworm disease, although PH has been described in association with a variety of congenital and acquired cardiopulmonary conditions, including pneumonia in young dogs, chronic tracheobronchial disease, and suspected interstitial lung disease (Johnson et al. 1999a, Pyle et al. 2004).

History and signalment

PH is a secondary condition and any age or breed can be affected. It seems to be recognized less commonly in cats than in dogs. Young animals with congenital cardiac shunts are at risk, and puppies with severe pneumonia can also develop PH. Adult animals with mitral insufficiency, cardiomyopathy, or chronic pulmonary disease can develop PH at any stage during the course of disease. A history of acute or chronic heartworm disease would indicate an increased risk for pulmonary vascular disease. Clinical signs and historical complaints generally reflect the underlying cardiac or pulmonary conditions; thus, the majority of animals have nonspecific complaints of cough, respiratory distress, or lethargy. Interestingly, syncope appears to be a relatively common finding.

Physical examination

Abnormalities on physical examination usually reflect cardiopulmonary pathology. Auscultation will reveal harsh crackles and wheezes with bronchitis, or fine crackles and tachycardia with pulmonary edema of heart failure. Murmurs of tricuspid or pulmonic insufficiency can be detected during systole or diastole respectively, when the right ventricle or pulmonary artery dilates to accommodate pressure overload on the right heart. The murmur of mitral insufficiency is common in animals with valvular insufficiency or cardiomyopathy, in the presence of absence of cardiac failure. A prominent second heart sound is occasionally heard as the pulmonic valve closes against elevated pressure. Animals may develop right heart failure from pulmonary hypertension and display jugular venous distention, ascites, or subcutaneous edema.

Diagnostic findings

Laboratory evaluation is directed toward identification of underlying disease conditions that may be associated with pulmonary hypertension. A minimum database and occult heartworm test are recommended when PH is suspected. Polycythemia could suggest chronic hypoxia as a risk factor for PH. Pulse oximetry or an arterial blood gas analysis would support hypoxemia or acidosis as factors contributing to PH. Additional diagnostic testing would be focused on identifying specific underlying conditions.

Chest radiographs show a variety of abnormalities in PH but none are pathognomonic for the condition. Cardiomegaly, particularly right ventricular enlargement, pulmonary infiltrates, and large pulmonary arteries are expected in animals with PH (Figure 8.6), although these changes are nonspecific. An electrocardiogram may reveal a right-axis deviation

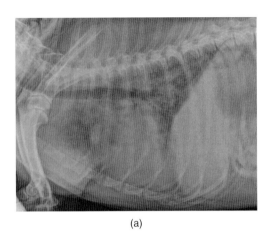
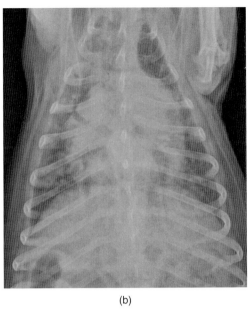

(a)   (b)

Figure 8.6. Right lateral (a) and dorsoventral (b) radiographs from a 13-year-old FS Terrier mix dog presented for tachypnea and collapse demonstrate diffuse, coalescing bronchoalveolar infiltrates throughout the lung region. There is mild right heart enlargement and a prominent main pulmonary artery bulge at 1:00. Doppler echocardiography revealed a pressure gradient of 70 mm Hg. Pulmonary hypertension in this case was secondary to interstitial fibrosis.

pattern (deep S waves in leads 1, 2, 3, and aVF) if right ventricular enlargement is severe, although detection of ECG changes is variable.

Doppler echocardiography can be used for noninvasive prediction of pulmonary artery pressure when a high-velocity regurgitant jet across the tricuspid or pulmonic valve is detected in the absence of pulmonic stenosis. Systolic or diastolic pulmonary artery pressure is estimated by application of the modified Bernoulli equation (the modified Bernoullie equation—Equation 8.1) to the maximal velocity of regurgitant flow across the tricuspid or pulmonic valve. A peak tricuspid regurgitant velocity ≥ 2.8 m/second estimates a systolic PAP ≥ 32 mm Hg (Figure 8.7) and a pulmonic insufficiency velocity ≥ 2.2 m/second estimates a diastolic PAP ≥ 20 mm Hg, suggesting PH. Right atrial pressure can be estimated clinically and added to the Doppler-derived pressure gradient to provide a closer approximation of pulmonary artery pressure.

$$\Delta P = 4 \times \left(\text{velocity}\right)^2 \qquad (8.1)$$

where ΔP is the right ventricular–right atrial pressure gradient when the velocity of tricuspid regurgitation is used and the right ventricular–pulmonary artery pressure gradient when pulmonic insufficiency is used. Velocity is in meters per second.

Subjective changes in echocardiographic parameters aid in the detection of PH. The main pulmonary artery is typically dilated, and a distinctive change is noted in the velocity profile of blood flow across the pulmonic valve with an increased rate of rise in pulmonary pressure. The deceleration phase can be rapid, or a delayed deceleration with mid-systolic notching is seen. Right ventricular dilatation and hypertrophy and right atrial enlargement

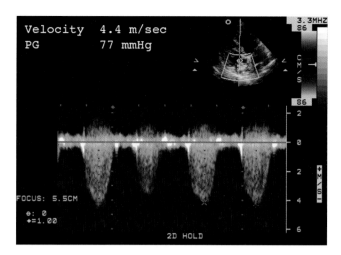

Figure 8.7. Doppler echocardiography from the dog depicted in Figure 8.6 reveals right ventricular hypertrophy, and mild tricuspid regurgitation with an instantaneous maximal velocity of 4.4 m/second (right ventricular–right atrial pressure gradient of 77 mm Hg).

can be encountered in dogs or cats diagnosed with PH, although severe right ventricular hypertrophy is uncommon in dogs that develop pulmonary hypertension when they are greater than 1 year of age. The left ventricle often appears small because of poor filling, and the interventricular septum is thick. Paradoxic septal motion suggests right ventricular pressure overload.

Definitive measurement of pulmonary artery pressure requires catheterization of the right heart with an end-hole Swan Ganz balloon-flotation catheter, although this is rarely done in clinical practice due to the need for sedation or general anesthesia.

Treatment

Treatment of the primary disease condition is essential for management of secondary pulmonary hypertension. Dogs or cats with chronic tracheobronchial disease may improve with theophylline treatment. Heart failure is first managed with diuretics and ACE inhibitors. Anticoagulant therapy is sometimes used to limit in situ thrombosis. Phosphodiesterase-5 (PDE-5) inhibitors, sildenafil, and tadalafil have been investigated as adjunct therapy for pulmonary hypertension. Inhibition of PDE-5 elevates cyclic GMP, a selective pulmonary vasodilator. Specific dosing regimens have not been established but sildenafil is often started at 0.5–2.0 mg/kg BID–TID. Echocardiographic monitoring for efficacy in reducing pulmonary pressure and blood pressure monitoring for hypotension should be performed, although studies have presented conflicting results on the effects of sildenafil on pulmonary artery pressure (Bach et al. 2006; Kellum and Stepien 2007).

Prognosis

It is unclear whether or how development of pulmonary hypertension might affect the prognosis of an animal with cardiopulmonary disease. In one retrospective study, the magnitude of elevation in pulmonary artery pressure had no direct impact on survival (Johnson et al. 1999a).

Noncardiogenic Pulmonary Edema and Acute Respiratory Distress Syndrome

Pathophysiology

Noncardiogenic pulmonary edema (NCPE) results from overexpansion of extracellular fluid volume due to intravenous fluid administration, decreased oncotic pressure, or from damage to the permeability of the alveolocapillary membrane. The most serious cause, permeability edema, causes protein-rich fluid to flood the alveoli. It can result from pulmonary insults including aspiration of gastric contents, severe upper airway obstruction, inhalant injury, and from extrapulmonary disorders such as sepsis, electric shock, central nervous system disease, pancreatitis, or disseminated intravascular coagulation (Drobatz et al. 1995). This condition can progress to acute respiratory distress syndrome (ARDS) with refractory hypoxemia, decreased pulmonary compliance, hyaline membrane formation, and ultimately respiratory failure.

History and signalment

NCPE should be considered in an animal with a history of a predisposing event that displays difficulty breathing or tachypnea. Any age, breed, or species can be affected.

Physical examination

Thoracic auscultation is expected to reveal tachypnea and bilateral, moist, and fine crackles. Detection of upper respiratory stridor in conjunction with such lower respiratory signs would suggest laryngeal paralysis or collapse as a cause for NCPE. Signs of systemic disease such as peripheral edema, neurologic signs, abdominal pain, or external burns are variably found depending on the cause of NCPE.

Diagnostic findings

Stress-induced hyperglycemia and a stress leukogram are common hematologic findings. Pulse oximetry or arterial blood gas will reflect poor oxygenation through decreased hemoglobin saturation with oxygen or hypoxemia with an increased alveolar–arterial oxygen gradient. Thoracic radiographs reveal bilateral symmetric infiltrates (typically alveolar) that are concentrated in the caudodorsal lung fields (Figure 8.8).

Treatment

Aggressive control of the primary disease process is essential for control of NCPE. Oxygen supplementation is indicated when tachypnea or labored respirations are noted, and generalized supportive care should be administered. Cautious intravenous fluid therapy should be provided because breakdown of the alveolocapillary membrane can result in fluid extravasation into the alveolus. Diuretics, positive inotropes, and corticosteroids have not been proven efficacious for specific treatment of noncardiogenic pulmonary edema, although they may be indicated to treat the primary disease process. Mechanical ventilation should be considered for patients with intractable respiratory difficulty.

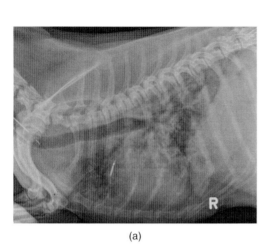
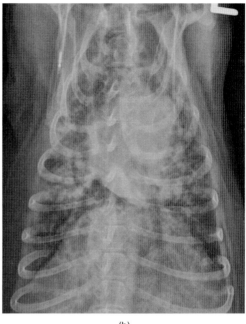

(a)   (b)

Figure 8.8. Right lateral (a) and dorsoventral (b) radiographs from a 10-year-old FS Dachshund show severe diffuse coalescing bronchoalveolar infiltrates. *Escherichia coli* bronchopneumonia progressing to ARDS was confirmed histologically in this dog by the presence of fibrin in the alveolar space, hyaline membrane formation, and type II pneumocyte hyperplasia.

Prognosis

Animals with fluid overload that have acceptable renal function usually respond to a decrease in supplemental fluids and diuretic therapy. A guarded prognosis should be offered for animals with NCPE due to suspected permeability edema, even when aggressive therapy is pursued. Survival to discharge for animals ventilated for therapy of ARDS was 10%, while 30% of animals mechanically ventilated for treatment of aspiration pneumonia survived (Hopper et al. 2007).

References

Alwood AJ, Downend AB, Brooks MB, et al. Anticoagulant effects of low-molecular-weight heparins in healthy cats. J Vet Int Med. 2007; 21: 378–387.

Bach JF, Rozanski EA, MacGregor J, et al. Retrospective evaluation of sildenafil citrate as a therapy for pulmonary hypertension in dogs. J Vet Int Med. 2006; 20: 1132–1135.

Bourque AC, Conboy G, Miller LM, Whitney H. Pathological findings in dogs naturally infected with Angiostrongylus vasorum in Newfoundland and Labrador, Canada. J Vet Diag Invest. 2008; 20: 11–20.

Browne LE, Carter TD, Levy JK, et al. Pulmonary arterial disease in cats seropositive for *Dirofilaria immitis* but lacking adult heartworms in the heart and lungs. Am J Vet Res. 2005; 66: 1544–1549.

Chapman PS, Boag AK, Guitan, Boswood A. Angiostrongylus vasorum infection in 23 dogs (1999–2002). J Small Animal Pract. 2004; 45: 435–440.

Drobatz KJ, Saunders HM, Pugh CR, Hendricks JC. Noncardiogenic pulmonary edema in dogs and cats: 26 cases (1987–1993). J Am Vet Med Assoc. 1995; 206: 1732–1736.

Glaus TM, Soldati G, Maurer R, Ehrensperger F. Clinical and pathological characterisation of primary pulmonary hypertension in a dog. Vet Records. 2004; 154: 786–789.

Hettlich BF, Ryan K, Bergman RL, et al. Neurologic complications after melarsomine dihydrochloride treatment for Dirofilaria immitis in three dogs. J Am Vet Med Assoc. 2003; 223: 1456–1461.

Hogan DF, Andrews DA, Green HW, et al. Antiplatelet effects and pharmacodynamics of clopidogrel in cats. J Am Vet Med Assoc. 2004; 225: 1406–1411.

Hopper K, Haskins SC, Kass PH, et al. Indications, management, and outcome of long-term positive pressure ventilation in dogs and cats: 148 cases (1990–2001). J Am Vet Med Assoc. 2007; 230: 64–75.

Johnson L, Boon J, Orton EC. Clinical characteristics of 53 dogs with Doppler-derived evidence of pulmonary hypertension: 1992–1996. J Vet Int Med 1999a; 13: 440–447.

Johnson LR, Lappin MR, Baker DC. Pulmonary thromboembolism in 29 dogs: 1985–1995. Vet Int Med. 1999b; 13: 338–345.

Kellum HB, Stepien RL. Sildenafil citrate therapy in 22 dogs with pulmonary hypertension. J Vet Int Med. 2007; 21: 1258–1264.

Liska WD, Poteet BA. Pulmonary embolism associated with canine total hip replacement. Vet Surg. 2003; 32: 178–186.

Litster A, Atkins C, Atwell R. Acute death in heartworm-infected cats: Unraveling the puzzle. Vet Parasitol. 2008; 158: 196–203.

Norris CR, Griffey SM, Samii VF. Pulmonary thromboembolism in cats: 29 cases (1987–1997). J Am Vet Med Assoc. 1999; 215: 1650–1654.

Pyle RL, Abbott J, MacLean H. Pulmonary hypertension and cardiovascular sequelae in 54 dogs. Int J Appl Res Vet Med. 2004; 2: 99–109.

Vargo CL, Taylor SM, Carr A, Jackson ML. The effect of a low molecular weight heparin on coagulation parameters in healthy cats. Can J Vet Res. 2009; 73: 132–136.

Venco L, Genchi C, Genchi M, et al. Clinical evolution and radiographic findings of feline heartworm infection in asymptomatic cats. Vet Parasitol. 2008; 158: 232–237.

Willesen JL, Kristensen AT, Jensen AL, et al. Efficacy and safety of imidacloprid/moxidectin spot-on solution and fenbendazole in the treatment of dogs naturally infected with Angiostrongylus vasorum (Baillet, 1866). Vet Parasitol. 2007; 147: 258–264.

Zabka TS, Campbell FE, Wilson DW. Pulmonary arteriopathy and idiopathic pulmonary arterial hypertension in six dogs. Vet Pathol. 2006; 43: 510–522.

Glossary

Alar fold: Lateral ridge at the external opening of the nostril

Arytenoid: Cartilage wings that form the lateral walls of the larynx

Bronchiectasis: Irreversible dilatation of the airways

Bronchitis: nonspecific airway inflammation

Bronchomalacia: Greater than 50% collapse of one or more primary or segmental bronchi.

Bronchoscopy: Endoscopic evaluation of the inner aspects of the airways, with a flexible or rigid, fiberoptic or videoendoscope

Bronchoalveolar lavage: Instillation and aspiration of warmed sterile saline into an isolated lung segment to retrieve airway fluid for culture and cytology

Carina: Vertical ridge of cartilage separating the left and right principal bronchi

Caval syndrome: Systemic illness, respiratory distress, liver or renal dysfunction, congestive heart failure, and/or DIC that occurs as a complication of heartworm disease

Chemosis: Swelling or edema of the conjunctiva. Can be associated with infection, inflammation, or fluid overload

Choana: One of the caudal openings of the nasal cavity into the nasopharynx (plural/choanae)

Chorioretinitis: Inflammation of the uveal tract of the eye, with the primary site in the vascular layer (choroid) and secondary inflammation in the neural layer (retina)

Ciliary dyskinesia: Defective ciliary motion, can be primary or secondary

Concha: Thin bones of the nose (turbinates; dorsal, ventral, and middle within the nasal cavity and the ethmoid system caudally)

Cranial vena cava syndrome: Edema of the head, neck, and front limbs due to obstruction of the cranial vena cava, often by a mediastinal mass

Cribriform plate: Bony separation between the nasal cavity and brain containing sieve-like perforations (part of the ethmoid bone)

Cyanosis: Bluish discoloration of mucous membranes indicating the presence of >5 g/dL of deoxygenated hemoglobin; may be central or peripheral.

Dynamic airway collapse: Excessive opening (on inspiration) and closing (on expiration) of airways beyond the carina; often a sign of bronchomalacia

Dysphagia: Difficulty eating or swallowing

Dysphonia: Abnormal vocalization or a change in meow or bark

Dyspnea: The sensation of difficult or uncomfortable breathing. This is a *symptom* described to physicians by the patient

Epistaxis: Hemorrhage from the nose

Ethmoid bone: The bony structure comprising the ethmoturbinates and the cribriform plate

Eupnea: Normal respiration

Extrathoracic: Refers to airways from the thoracic inlet to the nose

Hemoptysis: Coughing up blood

Hypercapnea/Hypercarbia: Increased arterial carbon dioxide content

Hyperpnea: Increased minute ventilation due to increased depth and/or rate of respiration

Hyperventilation: Increased alveolar ventilation in excess of CO_2 production

Hypoventilation: Decreased alveolar ventilation characterized by increased arterial P_aCO_2

Hypoxemia: Decreased arterial oxygen content (P_aO_2 < 80 mm Hg at sea level)

Intercostal: Between the ribs

Intrathoracic: Refers to airways within the chest cavity, beyond the thoracic inlet

Laryngeal saccules: Mucosal folds found within the laryngeal crypts between the vocal fold and the arytenoid

Meatus: Passageway within the nasal cavity between the conchal folds; dorsal, middle, ventral, and common

Mediastinum: Space within the central portion of the chest defined by the thoracic inlet cranially, the diaphragm caudally, the mediastinal pleura laterally, the paravertebral gutter and ribs dorsally, and the sternum ventrally. It contains the heart, great vessels, and esophagus and separates these structures from the left and right lung lobes. Fenestrae within the mediastinum allow communication between the two sides of the thorax in dogs and cats (incomplete mediastinum)

Naris: One of the external openings of the nasal cavity, i.e., nostril (plural/nares)

Nasopharynx: Region of the pharynx above the soft palate. Bounded rostrally by the choanae and extending caudally into the oropharynx, it allows passage of air during nasal breathing.

Oropharynx: Region of the pharynx between the soft palate, base of the tongue, and the epiglottis

P_aO_2: Partial pressure of arterial oxygen (mm Hg)

P_aCO_2: Partial pressure of arterial carbon dioxide (mm Hg)

Pleura: Serous membranes lining the thoracic wall (parietal pleura) and lungs (visceral pleura), responsible for producing and absorbing lubricating fluid within the pleural space

Pneumonia: Inflammation of the lung parenchyma

Retinochoroiditis: Inflammation of the uveal tract of the eye, with the primary site in the neural layer (retina) and secondary inflammation in the vascular layer (choroid)

Reverse sneeze: Repeated efforts to inspire against a closed glottis; usually occurs with the head in a raised position and is a sign of nasopharyngeal irritation.

Rhinoscopy: Endoscopic evaluation of the interior of the nasal cavity

SPO_2: Hemoglobin saturation with oxygen (%)

Staphylectomy: Soft palate resection

Stertor: Snoring or snorting sound due to soft tissue obstruction of the upper airway

Stridor: High-pitched inspiratory sound due to upper airway obstruction, typically within the larynx

Orthopnea: Inability to breathe in the supine position

Tachypnea: Rapid respiratory rate

Thoracic inlet: Site of transition between atmospheric and intrapleural pressure effects on the airway, located anatomically at the level of the first thoracic vertebrae and first pair of ribs

Tracheobronchomalacia: Tracheal collapse with concurrent collapse of 1 or more larger bronchi.

Tracheotomy: Incision into the trachea through the skin and cervical muscles

Tracheostomy: Creation of an opening into the trachea for insertion of a tube or for permanent respiration

Turbinate: Thin bones of the nose (concha; dorsal, ventral, and middle within the nasal cavity and the ethmoid system caudally)

Xeromycteria: Dry nose syndrome resulting from loss of parasympathetic stimulation of serous secretions from the lateral nasal gland.

Index